The College Student's Guide to

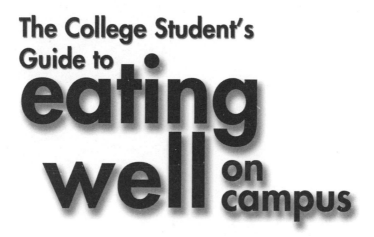

eating well on campus

The College Student's Guide to
eating well on campus

REVISED AND EXPANDED

Ann Selkowitz Litt, M.S., R.D., L.D.

Tulip Hill Press
Bethesda, Maryland

The College Student's Guide to Eating Well on Campus—2nd Edition
Copyright © 2005
by Ann Selkowitz Litt, M.S., R.D., L.D.
All rights reserved.

Published by
Tulip Hill Press
5257 River Road #305
Bethesda, MD 20816

ISBN 0-9700139-1-4

The nutrition advice appearing in this book is intended for use as a reference to help you make informed decisions about your diet and health. It is not a substitute for treatment that may have been prescribed by your doctor. You should consult with your doctor and obtain his or her approval before making any diet changes. The author disclaims any liability arising directly or indirectly from *The College Student's Guide to Eating Well on Campus.*

Nutrient analysis data contained in this book was obtained from sources including: *Bowes and Church's Food Values of Portions Commonly Used*, by Jean Pennington (J.B. Lippincott Company, 1994.) FoodWorks (The Nutrition Company, P.O. Box 447, Long Valley, NJ 07853) and various food companies. Data listed for several comparable foods may represent an average value. Menu items and nutritional data listed here are current as of publication. All brand-name products cited in this book are the registered trademark properties of their respective companies.

Publisher's Cataloging-in-Publication
(Provided by Quality Books, Inc.)

Litt, Ann.
    The college student's guide to eating well on campus / Ann Litt.
— 2nd ed.
        p.   cm.
    Includes index
    LCCN: 00–90701
    ISBN: 0–9700139–1–4
        1. Nutrition—Requirements.   2. College students—Nutrition.
    3. Cookery.   I. Title.
    RA784.L58   2000   613.2'088'379
                                                                QBI00–451

Contents

PART II

Weighing In

PART III

Challenges to Eating Well in College

Vegetarianism is a popular trend among college students. There are special nutritional considerations to be aware of if you choose a plant-based diet. Learn about:

- The various types of vegetarian diets
- Strategies for eating a well-balanced, healthy vegetarian diet
- Selecting vegetarian meals on campus

If you are a college athlete your nutritional needs may be different than non-athletic students. A recent study by The National Collegiate Athletic Association's (NCAA) also suggests that athletes are at an increased risk for developing an eating disorder. Find out:

- The nutritional needs of athletes
- How to choose pre and post-game meals
- The details on carbohydrate loading and other diet manipulations that may enhance performance

Most colleges are ready, willing and able to accommodate reasonable requests for following your special diet whether it is a diet for celiac disease, food allergies or even sulfite sensitivity. The keys to making the process successful are:

- Knowing your problem foods or diet modification
- Being familiar with special food products
- Learning who to approach in college dining services
- Approaching the correct person with requests in hand

Experimentation with alcohol, illicit drugs and prescribed medications can affect your nutritional status. Understand:

- What happens inside your body when you drink
- The impact of marijuana on your diet
- Dangerous drug/diet interactions
- Guidelines for moderating alcohol consumption

PART IV

College Cooking

List of Charts

Acknowledgments

Finishing a book, even "just" a new edition, is a group effort. I am so grateful to my family, friends, clients and colleagues who have helped me pull this together again. Special thanks go to:

Sue Moores, who is not only the best editor, she is a real friend. Thank you for once again making me look good.

Emily Greenberg and Lisa Weiss who were so incredibly helpful in collecting data for this new edition.

Barry Kerrigan and his group at Desktop Miracles, for hanging in there with me and delivering a terrific product.

Those college students who are my clients and those who just hang around my kitchen. You make what I do for a living seem worthwhile.

Sodexho Food Service for allowing me to spend so much time on your campuses and see campus eating in a whole new light.

Marsha Hudnall, M.S., R.D., Theresa Anderson, R.D., Monika Woolsey, M.S., R.D. and Shelley Case, R.D. for your expertise and wisdom in helping me shape the new chapters.

The college based dietitians who share so generously on your listserv. You do an outstanding job.

My sons, David and Jordan, who have allowed me to peak into their campus refrigerators (don't ask!) and their college lives to learn more than I really need to know about how college students eat.

My mother, who to this day asks her nutritionist/adult/daughter what she is having for dinner.

And my husband, Dan, my editor, coach, and the best college roommate. I could never do this without you.

For Dan, David
and Jordan

Preface

What's new in college eating since the release of the first edition of **The College Student's Guide to Eating Well on Campus** in 2000? A lot! Forget institutionalized dining halls and cafeteria lines. Campus meals have gone mainstream. Sushi, lattes and paninis are on the menu, making it seem more like you're eating in a trendy downtown area than the college dining hall. This updated version incorporates the changes I've seen in campus eating when visiting colleges, reflects general health concerns affecting college age students and provides the information that you—the college student—has requested.

Some schools and their student populations care a lot about the type of food offered and others continue to relegate nutrition to a low priority. Regardless of where nutrition stacks up on your campus, college students want it all—the healthy sandwich bars and the 24-hour "wings to go" delivery for those late-night munchies. **Eating Well on Campus** is your guide to balance—making the best choices from what's available to you.

Since the first edition was released in 2000, health reports point to a dramatic change in the incidence of obesity and diet-related problems—even among college age students. College students have responded by dieting. Because I believe restrictive dieting does more harm than good, I avoided the whole topic of dieting in the first edition. This time, I didn't want to miss an opportunity to help you deal with this problem—or perhaps avoid it. A new chapter, **Reality Dieting,** presents the ins and outs of popular diets so you can make informed decisions.

Another new chapter, **Special Requests,** is included to help those students who arrive on campus with food issues such as food allergies, celiac disease or hypoglycemia. College foodservices are ready and willing to accommodate your reasonable requests. Use this chapter to assist you in managing these problems away from home.

We have a new food guidance system, MyPyramid, and tools to make that useful to you are included in this new edition. New and popular food chains have made their homes near campuses. **Chapter 2** has been updated to include nutritional analysis on these eateries.

The biggest change since the first edition of **Eating Well on Campus** debuted in 2000 is that my own children headed off to college and I was able to view college eating not only through the eyes of my clients—but up close and personal! This has broadened my appreciation for college eating and has given me a greater understanding of the challenges students face.

The bottom line about college eating is there are options galore on most campuses. You might get bored with what is offered (but hey— how many times do you order the same exact item in a restaurant?) and you might long for your familiar brand of yogurt. If you can organize your schedules, get some regular exercise and learn how to balance the choices available, **Eating Well on Campus** can help you graduate with your health intact and maybe even a greater appreciation for eating well. Bon Appetit.

PART I
Nutrition 101

1

Feeding Your Body

You are what you eat." Not a news flash, but newsworthy. What you eat influences how you look, how you feel, and how you perform mentally (on tests and exams) and physically (in energy level and sports). What you eat even affects how you sleep at night. To look good, feel good, and perform well, you need to eat well, which means taking the only body you have and feeding it so it's the best it can possibly be.

Besides making you look and feel good, eating well can help prevent chronic problems like heart disease, cancer, osteoporosis, high blood pressure, and diabetes. Who cares? Those kinds of problems are light-years away—health hazards for older people right? Well . . . sort of. You're young, healthy, and chances are you would like to keep it that way.

Eating well today means living well tomorrow—literally. What you choose to eat ultimately impacts your long-term health, but what you ate this morning or what you have for dinner tonight has immediate repercussions. Take a look at your mood, your stamina, yourself in the mirror; food is an important factor in each of these.

It's fairly easy to eat well. It doesn't have to cost a lot of money, and you don't have to rack your brain over how to do it. Although headlines in newspapers and magazines and information on the Web may lead you to believe you have to micromanage your way to better health, all you really need is a good dose of common sense and an open mind to try new things.

In the interest of staying healthy, take the quiz in Chart 1–1 to see if you eat well and if you know how nutrition affects your health.

Whether you have a knack for nutrition or need a little guidance, you'll find great tips and ideas in the pages that follow. Read on for the simple, yet significant facts you should know about the food you eat.

Nutrition Know-How

Get smart about food. There are no good foods or bad foods, but there are some foods that are better than others because they contain nutrients in addition to calories. Foods that have lots of calories but few nutrients have earned the title of "junk food." Your job is to focus on the better foods, the ones that contain more nutrients (see Chart 1–2).

Besides choosing health-promoting foods, eating well is also about balance—balancing healthy food choices with less than healthy ones. The goal of eating well is not about swearing off junk food—it's about letting the healthy stuff prevail. If you do, chances are you'll feel better because you are eating better.

Eating Well: The Big Picture

The foods you eat need to satisfy you when you're hungry, taste good, be affordable, and ideally give your body two things: energy and **nutrients**.

CHART 1-1

Are You Nutrition Savvy? True or False

1. A healthy diet includes some junk food.
2. It's impossible for college students to eat well on campus.
3. If you have a bakery bagel for breakfast, you've just eaten about four servings of grain foods.
4. Eating well affects how you feel.
5. Eating breakfast can help control late night binges.
6. Natural foods are healthier than other foods.
7. You need to eliminate pasta from your diet to lose weight.
8. Vitamins provide you with extra energy.
9. Eating 5–6 meals a day is the best meal pattern for a college student.
10. Eating well today is important in preventing heart disease, cancer, osteoporosis, and diabetes.

Answers

1. **True.** Eating well is about balance. Choose foods from the grain group, fruit and veggies group, dairy and protein group . . . and then some that don't fit in anywhere, but you eat them because they taste good, not because they are good for you.
2. **False.** Although college students can easily eat a poor diet, they can just as easilty eat a healthy diet. Read on for details.
3. **True.** Bakery bagels are quite large and generally contain between 250–350 calories per serving which translates into four to five servings of grain foods.
4. **True.** You are, quite literally, what you eat. A well-balanced diet will give you more energy, protect you from illness, and probably make you look better.
5. **True.** Research suggests that breakfast eaters tend to weigh less and have better balance to their day. College students should plan to eat a snack if they are up late at night, but it should be real food as opposed to unlimited amounts of "junk".
6. **False.** While natural may be healthy, it does not have much to do with the nutrients in a food.
7. **False.** Losing weight is about portions and calories. No one particular food contributes to excess weight. If you eat a reasonable amount of pasta it is fine to include in your diet . . . even if you are trying to lose weight.
8. **False.** Vitamins to not contain calories, nor do they increase your energy. A diet rich in natural vitamins and good wholesome food is the best way to feel energized.
9. **False.** There isn't a best pattern. The number of meals you eat and when you eat them should fit your schedule. If you are a late night person, be sure to eat a late night snack.
10. **True.** Many of the chronic diseases affecting adults are diet-related. Eating a healthy diet can prevent or delay the onset of some of these conditions.

CHART 1–2

Nutritious or Not?

Those foods in bold contain calories and nutrients. The others may taste good and are fine to eat occasionally, but they are more appropriately called junk food because they supply mainly calories and taste . . . and few nutrients.

	CALORIES	PROTEIN (gm)	FAT (gm)	CHO	FIBER (gm)	CALCIUM (mg)
Skim milk (8 oz.)	80	8	0	10	–	300
Coca-Cola (12 oz.)	140	0	0	27	–	0
Apple	80	–	0	21	3	–
Apple pie (small slice)	210	–	9	29	0	–
Pop Tart	210	2	6	37	0	–
Whole wheat toast (2 slices)	120	6	1	23	3	–
Grilled Chicken Sandwich	280	25	7	29	1	80
Big Mac	560	25	30	46	3	25
Donut and coffee	230	2	12	30	–	–
Cereal/skim milk	150	7	–	28	5	150

(–) Indicates it isn't a significant source of this nutrient or data is unavailable.

Nutrients can be divided into two categories: "big" nutrients, called **macronutrients**, and "smaller" ones (though no less important), called **micronutrients.** Macronutrients are **carbohydrate**, **protein**, and **fat**. They are digested and used by your body for fuel or energy and do certain jobs in your body, such as building new cells, transporting vitamins in the blood, and causing important chemical reactions to occur inside your body.

The amount of energy produced when a food is digested is measured in **calories**.

Calories are your body's source of fuel. You burn calories all the time: in class, when you work out, even while you sleep. Nearly every food contains at least some calories (more about this in Chapter 6). If you eat more calories than your body burns, you gain weight. If you eat fewer calories than your body needs, you lose weight, but, at the same time, you may be depriving yourself of necessary energy and important health-promoting nutrients (more about this in Chapter 8).

Proportion Your Portions: Carbohydrates, Protein, and Fat

About 50 to 60 percent of your calories should include foods rich in carbohydrates, such as breads, cereals, rice, and pasta. Ten to 20 percent should come from protein-rich foods, such as meat, dairy products, and legumes. The remaining 20 to 30 percent of your calories can come from that tasty stuff called fat (see Chart 1–3).

Carbohydrates

There are two types of carbohydrates: **simple** and **complex**. Carbohydrates are made up of small units of sugar linked together (see Chart 1–4). The difference between simple and complex carbohydrates is based on how many units of sugar are linked together—the more units, the more complex the carbohydrate.

Simple carbohydrates are found in foods that taste sweet, such as **soft drinks, cookies, candy,** and **fruit**. They are easy to digest and often give you a quick burst of energy. **Complex carbohydrates**, also referred to as "starch," are found in **pasta, bread, potatoes, rice, cereal, legumes** and to a lesser extent, **veggies**. They take longer to digest and provide a more even flow of energy to the body.

CHART 1–3

Calorie Distribution for a Typical Day

BREAKFAST
1 cup Shredded Wheat
1 banana
1 cup skim milk
1 slice whole wheat toast/
margarine

LUNCH
Vegetable soup
PB & J sandwich
Apple
2 cookies
1 cup skim milk

SNACK
Frozen yogurt cone

DINNER
Chicken breast
Baked potato
Broccoli

SNACK
1 slice pizza

CHART 1–4

Learning about Carbs*

There are three different types of carbohydrates, all or which are made up of units of sugar.

- **Simple carbohydrates** are composed of one or two units of "sugar." Simple sugars taste sweet. A simple carbohydrate with one unit of sugar is called a monosaccharide. (mono=one, saccharide=sugar). Examples of monosaccharides are:

    Fructose or "fruit sugar"
    Galactose
    Glucose or "blood sugar"
    A carbohydrate with two units of sugar is called a disaccharide (di=two). Examples of disaccharides are:

    Sucrose or "table sugar" = glucose + fructose
    Lactose or "milk sugar" = glucose + galactose
    Maltose or "malt sugar" = glucose + glucose

- **Complex carbohydrates** are composed of many units of sugar. They are also known as polysaccharides (poly=many). Starch, found in potatoes, rice, and pasta, is an example of a polysaccharide.

- **Fiber** is a polysaccharide. It is different from starch because the bonds that link the sugar units together can't be digested or absorbed by our bodies. Fiber, therefore, is a carbohydrate that doesn't give us energy or calories.

- **Net impact carbs** is a term used by food companies marketing products to those following a low carb diet. Carbohydrates from wheat are replaced with fiber, sugar, alcohols, fat or soy flour. Net carbs supposedly have less impact on blood sugar but they still contain calories.

*Carbohydrates are abbreviated as CHO throughout the book.

Your body prefers carbohydrates for its fuel. When you eat carbo-rich foods, they are digested and broken down to glucose, which is then circulated in your blood to be used for fuel by every cell. What isn't used initially is converted to the storage form of carbohydrate, glycogen, and a small amount is stored in your muscles and liver. This is especially important in the athlete's diet (more on this in Chapter 9).

Sugar often gets a bad rap. Its sweet taste makes food taste good. Sugar-laden foods don't usually provide many other nutrients, however.

CHART 1–5

The Sweet Truth about Sugar and Sugar Substitutes

Sugar, that stuff that tastes so good, has received an undeserved bad rap. While sugar-laden products often provide little nutritional value, they aren't necessarily the culprits in disease either.

- **Sugar high.** Perhaps as a little kid, you weren't allowed to eat sugary things because it made you "hyper." There isn't any good data to support this.
- **Hypoglycemia.** A condition, not a disease, caused by a drop in your blood sugar. Sugar doesn't cause the problem, but you may need professional guidance about how to include sugar-rich foods in your diet so you don't feel the symptoms of hypoglycemia.
- **Cavities.** Tooth decay is a result of many things, not just a diet high in sugar. Carbohydrates play a part, but genetics and frequency of meals do also. Eating constantly and having foods like "sucking candy" in your mouth keeps the bacteria ripe for action.
- **Addiction.** Having a sweet tooth is quite different from an addiction. Sugary foods are often delicious, and controlling their intake can be a challenge. If you see them as "no-no" foods, their appeal is even greater. An actual addiction to sugar is difficult to document.

What about sugar substitutes?

Four approved sugar substitutes are used in our food supply: Saccharin (Sweet & Low®), Acesulfame K (Sunett™), Aspartame (Equal® or Nutrasweet®), and Sucralose (Splenda®). Their safety and usefulness has been hotly debated for years. Large amounts of saccharin have been shown to cause cancer in laboratory animals, but it's never been documented in humans. Aspartame can be harmful to people with a metabolic disorder known as PKU and may cause headaches in some. To date, acesulfame and sucralose appear to be safe.

Artificial sweeteners are helpful to people with diabetes because they often need to avoid sugar. But most use the no-calorie substitutes to cut calories. Unfortunately, replacing calories with artificial sweeteners doesn't seem to help much. Most users end up eating more calories than are saved by the "diet" product.

Dietary guidelines say, "sugar should be used in moderation." Sixteen calories per teaspoon seems like a meager amount to give up for enjoying the taste of something real. Although a diet cola here or there is probably not harmful for most people, it makes sense to enjoy moderate amounts of sugar if you want something sweet.

But that doesn't mean they can't be part of a healthy diet. They just need to be included in a minor way, to make sure there's room for all of the nutrient-rich foods your body needs. To help you separate fact from fiction, see Chart 1–5.

Fiber is considered a carbohydrate; however, your body cannot digest or absorb it, and it doesn't contain any calories (see Chart 1–6). There are two types of fiber: *soluble* and *insoluble*. *Soluble fiber* includes *oat bran, oatmeal, beans, peas, lentils, nuts, seeds, rice bran, barley, citrus*

CHART 1–6

Good Sources of Fiber*

Food	Serving	Fiber (gm)
Breads and Grains		
Whole wheat bread	2 slices	2-5
Bran muffin	1	2
Brown rice	1 cup, cooked	3
Cereals		
Fiber One	½ cup	13
100% Bran	½ cup	10
Bran Flakes	¾ cup	5
Raisin Bran	¾ cup	4.5
Special K	1 cup	1
Oatmeal (instant)	1 packet	2
Legumes		
Pinto beans	½ cup, cooked	6
Kidney beans	½ cup, cooked	4
Chickpeas	½ cup, cooked	4
Black beans	½ cup, cooked	3.5
Vegetables		
Broccoli	½ cup, cooked	3.5
Baked potato (with skin)	1 small	2.5
Baby carrots	5	3
Iceberg lettuce	1 cup	1
Fruit		
Apple	1	3
Pear	1	4.5
Strawberries	1 cup	2.5

*Always start gradually when increasing fiber—drink more fluids, preferably water. This allows the fiber to make its way through your body, alleviating constipation in the process.

fruits, strawberries and *apple pulp. Insoluble fiber* is found in *wheat bran, vegetables* and *whole grain breads* and *cereals.* Insoluble fiber helps move food through your digestive tract, regulates normal bowel movements and prevents constipation. It has been fondly termed by some nutrition experts as "the body's broom." Soluble fiber appears to help lower blood cholesterol. Because of these properties, eating a high fiber diet has been linked to decreased risk of certain diseases including heart disease and intestinal cancer.

Protein

Protein literally means "of prime importance." In a nutshell, it is. Bones, skin, hair, muscle, and organs are all made up of protein. Protein is responsible for many functions that keep the body strong, such as fighting infections, regulating body functions like blood sugar/ energy levels, and just plain keeping your body tissues, such as your skin, healthy.

Like carbohydrates, protein is made up of smaller units or building blocks called **amino acids**. Your body needs a combination of 20 different **amino acids** to perform its functions. While the body can produce 11 of the 20, it can't produce the rest. These nine are called **essential amino acids**, meaning you have to get them from the food you eat.

Many foods are rich in protein. Animal foods such as eggs, dairy products, meat, fish and poultry contain all of the essential amino acids your body needs. Plant based foods such as legumes, grains, vegetables and seeds contain protein, too, but the protein may be less concentrated because the amino acid patterns vary. A diet based on vegetable protein can still be nutritionally adequate. (see Chapter 8).

Fat

There exists a phobia about fat in food, but fat has important functions in the body and should be part of a healthy diet. Your body uses dietary fat, the fat you get from food, for invisible jobs, such as absorbing essential fat-soluble vitamins, protecting your organs from damage when you fall, and providing ready energy on demand (see Chart 1–7).

CHART 1–7

Fat in Food

Visible fat: oil salad dressing, mayonnaise, gravy, butter, margarine, dips
Less-visible fat: whole milk, cheese, skin on poultry, fast food burgers, chocolate candy, baked goods, chips, certain cuts of meat

Fat also provides "padding," which insulates you from the cold and protects your bones from breaking. Too much fat, however, is bad news. A diet high in fat is considered a contributing factor to obesity, heart disease, and cancer. You don't have to banish fat from your diet—but you do have to balance it—20 to 30 percent of your caloric intake, no more.

There are different types of fat: saturated fat, mono-unsaturated fat, polyunsaturated fat, trans-fatty acids, omega-3 fatty acids, and more (see Chart 1–8). Though some fats are considered to be less harmful to your body, others are touted as more beneficial. But too much of any kind of fat is no good. The best bet for a healthy diet is to keep all types of fat in check, which means no more than 20 to 30 percent of the calories you eat can come from fat.

Cholesterol has been a headline-grabber for years, and the press it's been getting is less than favorable. What exactly is cholesterol? It's a fat-like substance used by your body to form important substances such as vitamin D and those all-important sex-related hormones . . . estrogen and testosterone. Cholesterol doesn't contain any calories. It is found only in foods that come from animals. Amazingly, your liver is able to make nearly all the cholesterol your body needs. In short, it's pretty difficult for you to run low on cholesterol.

CHART 1–8

Know Your Fats

Cholesterol:

Not a fat at all, but a fat-like substance. Dietary cholesterol is found only in foods of animal origin: egg yolks, organ meats and whole milk dairy products. Blood cholesterol is a waxy substance in our body. It does occur naturally in our bodies. Certain people may be more prone to higher amounts of blood cholesterol, and certain people may produce more as a result of diet and lifestyle.

Saturated fats:

Saturated fats are found mostly in animal products such as whole milk dairy products, animal fat and vegetable products such as coconut oil, palm oil and palm kernel oils. They are considered "bad" because in large amounts they are the fats most likely responsible for raising your blood cholesterol.

Trans fats and hydrogenated fats:

During food processing when liquid vegetable oils are heated in the presence of hydrogen they become hydrogenated. This is how trans fatty acids are made. The more hydrogenated an oil, the harder it will be at room temperature. Trans fats are found in stick margarine, shortening and many commercially prepared baked goods, snack foods and processed foods. Trans fats are considered "bad" because they raise LDL cholesterol and lower HDL cholesterol.

Polyunsaturated and monounsaturated fats:

These fats are found primarily in oils from plants. Sunflower, safflower, corn and soybean bean oils are rich in polyunsaturated fats. Canola, olive and peanut oils, olives, avocados and nuts are rich in monounsaturated fats. They are considered "good" oils because they tend to decrease LDL levels and increase HDL levels. However, if you are overweight, keep in mind that all oils are high in calories so should be used carefully.

A Sample Chart of the Fat, Cholesterol and Calorie in Foods

FOOD	TOTAL FAT (gm)	CHOLESTEROL (mg)	CALORIES
Skim milk 8 oz.	trace	4	80
Whole milk 8 oz.	8	33	150
Cheese 1 oz.	9	29	115
Egg 1 whole	5	213	80
Lean beef 3 oz.	4	59	105
Chicken (no skin)	6	75	160
Tuna (water) 3oz.	1	25	115
Peanut butter 1 Tbs.	8	0	90
Avocado ½	15	0	160
Apple	trace	0	80
Butter	12	31	100
Margarine	12	0	100
Olive oil	14	0	120

Eating too much cholesterol has been linked to a higher risk for heart disease. But, unless you eat a lot of **egg yolks** or **liver**, or huge amounts of **meat** or **cheese**, chances of a cholesterol overdose are fairly remote.

Vitamins and Mineral

Vitamins and minerals are **micronutrients**, small but plenty powerful. Scientists have identified 13 vitamins and 22 minerals that are essential to good health, all of which are found in food. Vitamins are responsible for growth, regulating the energy you get from food, and protecting you from disease. Minerals are building blocks for bones; they help your muscles contract, your nerves respond to messages

---

CHART 1-9

The Alphabet Soup of Diet Standards

The Recommended Dietary Allowances (RDAs) have been used as a standard for planning diets since 1941. The **Dietary Reference Intakes (DRIs)** have been developed to expand and replace the RDAs. The DRIs represent a shift in emphasis from preventing deficiency diseases to decreasing the risk of chronic disease through nutrition. The DRIs are actually a set of four reference values:

Estimated Average Requirement (EAR): This is a nutrient intake value that is necessary to meet the estimated requirement of one-half of all healthy individuals in the population.

Adequate Intake (AI): The value set as a goal for an individual intake for nutrients that do not have a RDA.

Tolerable Upper Intake Level (UL): the highest level of a nutrient that is likely to pose no risk of adverse health effects to 98% of the population.

RDAs: the average daily dietary intake level of a nutrient that prevents deficiency in 98% of the population.

What appears on your food label? The **Reference Daily Intakes (RDI)**, which includes the recommended amounts of 19 vitamins, minerals and micronutrients and the **Daily Reference Values (DRV)** which is the recommended amounts of macronutrients: fat, fiber, carbohydrates, sodium, potassium and protein. The RDIs and the DRVs make the **Daily Values (DV)** and that is what appears on food labels.

from your brain, and initiate some of the chemical reactions that occur in your body (see Charts 1–9 & 1–10).

The perceived "nutritional protection" you get from taking a multivitamin supplement is not harmful, neither is it a fix for poor eating habits. Vitamins and minerals work together in the body. For example, vitamin C is helpful in absorbing the iron found in food; too little vitamin D makes calcium less absorbable; too much zinc can affect copper levels in your body. The list of interactions between vitamins and minerals is lengthy. Too much of one vitamin or mineral can upset the balance of others.

Food provides your body with a natural balance of vitamins and minerals and it delivers them in a form that is easier for your body to absorb. In other words, when it comes to eating well, "food first" is a refrain worth remembering. Certain situations may increase your need for a specific nutrient (see Chart 1–11). A visit to a Registered Dietitian

---

CHART 1–10

Vitamins and Minerals

Fat-soluble vitamins: **Vitamins A, D, E,** and **K** are called "fat soluble" since they don't dissolve in water. They can be stored in the body's fat, so we don't need to eat them every day. Although it's difficult to "overdose" on the vitamins when they occur naturally in food, taking large doses of fat-soluble vitamins can be toxic.

Water-soluble vitamins: The **B vitamins (thiamin, riboflavin, niacin, B6, B12, folic acid, pantothenic acid,** and **biotin), choline,** and **vitamin C** are "water soluble" since they can dissolve easily in water. They're not stored in the body, so there's a greater chance of being deficient if adequate amounts are not eaten regularly. Excess amounts of these vitamins are generally lost when you urinate.

Minerals: Our bodies require at least 22 minerals to "make things happen." We need larger amounts of **major minerals (calcium, chloride, magnesium, phosphorus, potassium, sodium,** and **sulfur)** than **trace minerals (arsenic, boron, chromium, cobalt, copper, fluoride, iodine, iron, manganese, molybdenum, nickel, selenium, silicon,** and **zinc).** Don't be fooled by the amounts required. The job of trace minerals is equally important. (Some of these minerals are not listed below, since we don't know enough about them.)

VITAMIN	WHAT IT DOES	GOOD FOOD SOURCES	RECOMMENDED AMOUNTS*
Vitamin A	Important for vision and immune system	Fortified milk, eggs, carrots, dark green leafy vegetables (vitamin A can be converted from beta-carotene, which is found in the body)	female: 800 mcg RE or 4,000 IU male: 1,000 mcg RE or 5,000 IU can be toxic above 25,000 IU
Vitamin D	Helps calcium absorption, important in bone formation	Fortified milk, egg yolks, fish oils (can be made by the body when skin is exposed to the sun)	5 mcg (200 IU)
Vitamin E	Antioxidant*	Vegetable oils, wheat germ, nuts	female: 8 mg or 12 IU male: 10 mg or 15 IU
Vitamin K	Important for blood clotting	Dark green leafy vegetables (can by made from body's own intestinal bacteria)	female (19-24): 60 mcg (25+): 65 mcg male (19-24): 70 mcg (25+): 80 mcg
Vitamin B1 (Thiamin)	Needed to metabolize carbohydrates for energy	Whole grain and enriched products (cereal, bread, pastas and rice) pork, legumes	female (14-18): 1 mg (19+): 1.1 mg male: 1.2 mg
Vitamin B2 (Riboflavin)	Needed to metabolize food for energy; Helps maintain skin and vision healthy	Whole grain and enriched products, dairy products, dark green leafy vegetables	female (14-18): 1.0 mg (19+): 1.1 mg male: 1.3 mg
Niacin (Vitamin B3)	Needed to metabolize food for energy; Helps maintain healthy skin	Meat, fish, poultry, eggs, milk, nuts, whole grain, cnd enriched products	female: 14 mg male: 16 mg
Vitamin B6 (Pyridoxine)	Helps the body make protein; Helps regulate the nervous system and regenerate red blood cells	Meat, fish, poultry, eggs, soybeans, nuts, whole grain breads and cereal	female (14-18): 1.2–1.5 mg (19+): 1.3–1.7 mg male: 1.3 mg
Vitamin B12	Needed to make red blood cells; involved in synthesis of DNA	Found only in foods of animal origin, including milk and eggs; fortified soy products may contain B12	2.4 mg
Folic Acid	Needed to make DNA and in formation of new cells	Dark green vegetables, orange juice legumes, whole grain, and enriched products	400 mcg
Biotin	Helps to metabolize food for energy	Widespread in food	14-18: 25 mcg 19+: 30 mcg

VITAMIN	WHAT IT DOES	GOOD FOOD SOURCES	RECOMMENDED AMOUNTS*
Pantothenic Acid	Helps to metabolize food for energy	Widespread in food	5 mg
Choline	Helps maintain normal liver function	Widespread in food	female (14-18): 400 mg (19+): 425 mg male: 450 mg
Vitamin C	Antioxidant; Helps fight infections promotes wound healing, and helps iron absorption	Oranges, grapefruit, berries, broccoli, tomatoes, potatoes, melons	60 mg
Calcium	Important in building and maintaining bone; Helps with muscle contracting, maintaining, normal nerve function, and blood clotting	Milk and milk products, broccoli, canned salmon and kale, sardines, calcium-fortified products such as orange juice and soy milk	14-18: 1300 mg 19+: 1000 mg
Chloride	Regulates fluids in the body	Table salt	750 mg
Magnesium	Important in building bone and regulating many body functions	Whole grains, legumes, nuts, dark green leafy vegetables	female (14-18): 360 mg (19+): 310 mg male (14-18): 410 mg (19+): 400 mg
Phosphorous	Important in building and maintaining bone; Necessary for metabolizing food	Widespread in food	14-18: 1250 mg 19+: 700 mg
Potassium	Helps regulate fluid and mineral balance and maintain normal blood pressure	bananas, melons, oranges, grapefruit, dried fruit, tomatoes meat, poultry and fish	not established
Sodium	Helps regulate fluid and mineral balance, regulates blood pressure	processed food	not established
Chromium	Works with insulin to help the body use blood sugar	meat, whole grains, nuts and seeds	50-200 mg
Copper	Important in hemo- globin formation Part of many enzymes	seafood, organ meats, nuts and seeds	1.5–3 mg
Fluoride	Protects teeth from decay	canned salmon, fluoridated water	female: 3 mg male (14-18): 3 mg 19+: 4 mg

VITAMIN	WHAT IT DOES	GOOD FOOD SOURCES	RECOMMENDED AMOUNTS*
Iodine	Important in thyroid hormone which regulates energy used by the body	saltwater fish, food grown near the coasts	150 mg
Iron	Needed to form hemoglobin meat, poultry, fish, legumes which is used to carry oxygen through the body	dried fruit, spinach, iron-fortified cereal	female: 15 mg male(14-18): 12 mg 19+: 10 mg
Manganese	Part of every enzyme	whole grain bread and cereal	2–5 mg
Molybdenum	Involved in red blood cell synthesis and enzyme and cereal functions	milk, legumes, whole grain breads	75–250 mcg
Selenium	Antioxidant	seafood, whole grain breads and seeds	female (15-18): 50 mcg 19+: 55 mcg male (15-18): 50 mcg 19+: 70 mcg
Zinc	Essential for growth Helps in wound healing	meat, seafood, whole grain bread and cereal, legumes, soy	female: 15 mg male: 10 mg

*These amounts are based on the current RDA or DRI's.

**Some vitamins and minerals function as antioxidants. An antioxidant stops certain toxic substances from building up in the body.

can help you plan a healthy diet, one that doesn't require supplements or at least one that uses them effectively. If you choose to take a supplement, be sure you know what it can and can't do, and get the most for your money (see Chart 1–12).

Herbal Relief

What about the raging market of herbal supplement—echinacea, St. John's Wort, gingko biloba, etc.? Even though more and more Americans are shelling out big money for these products, the quality and effectiveness of herbal supplements vary greatly, and in some cases, have yet to be proven.

The appeal of herbal supplements is that they are "natural," which can be interpreted as meaning safe and good, and, unlike medicine, they don't require a doctor's appointment for a prescription. Herbal supplements, or any supplement for that matter, appear to be a quick and effortless fix to problems that plague you, such as depression or fatigue. Quick fixes in health are few and far between and should be approached with caution. Herbal supplements need much more scientific documentation before they can be considered safe and helpful.

CHART 1–11

Do You Need a Supplement?

Certain situations require a closer look at specific nutrients in your diet. Although diet may do the trick, you might need a supplement to cover your bases. Just remember that supplements never correct a lousy diet.

- **Are you a smoker?** Along with all of the bad stuff smoking does to your body, it robs it of vitamin C. You need more, at least 100 mg more a day. This is easy to get by drinking orange juice or eating broccoli or strawberries. If these foods are not usually in your diet, consider a supplement.
- **Are you a strict vegetarian?** Unless you choose carefully, your diet can be deficient in certain nutrients (see Chapter 8).
- **Are you taking oral contraceptive agents (OCAs)?** Some preliminary research suggests your B6 level needs to be monitored because taking an OCA may increase your need for this vitamin. However, since large amounts can be dangerous, think food first before automatically supplementing.
- **Do you suffer from PMS?** Again, the research isn't conclusive, but eating a diet rich in calcium and B6 can alleviate the symptoms.
- **Are you catching a cold?** The role of large doses of vitamin C in preventing colds has been debated for years. What seems do be the current party line is that higher doses (>1500 mg) may decrease the severity and duration of a cold, but the research doesn't support using mega-doses to prevent a cold.
- **Feeling fatigued or stressed?** What student isn't? A strong dose of healthy eating and a good night's sleep is the best remedy. Vitamins do play a role in stress inflicted on your body, such as when wounds are healing or you're recovering from a broken bone. However, there is little to substantiate the need for extra vitamins to cope with emotional stress.

CHART 1–12

Tips for Choosing a Supplement

- **You don't get what you pay for**. Natural or synthetic generally doesn't matter, because your body can't recognize whether the supplement was manufactured in a lab or came from a natural source. For most supplements, it doesn't matter whether you buy a store brand, name brand, or natural. The only differences may be the ingredients added for taste, the packaging, and the price.
- **Check the expiration date**. Vitamins do lose their potency, so buy the one with the longest shelf life.
- **One hundred percent is enough**. Since it's possible to get toxic amounts of some vitamins and minerals, play it safe and stay with those that are about 100 percent of the standard. More is not better and may actually be unsafe for certain vitamins, such as vitamin A, calcium, folic acid, or vitamin D.
- **Choose a vitamin/mineral combo**. That way you can avoid disturbing the delicate balance that makes vitamins and minerals work best. In certain situations, you may need more than a standard supplement provides.
- **Timing is important**. It's best to take your supplement with meals. If you're taking a multivitamin with iron, don't take extra calcium at the same time, since high doses of calcium interfere with your ability to absorb iron.
- **Food first**. All of the expensive supplements in the store won't replace a healthy diet.

Many of the herbal supplements available have neither been adequately tested to substantiate the claims their sellers make, nor have they been tested to ensure that the ingredients in them are what they say they are. It is even unclear whether the ingredients listed are "biologically active," meaning that the supplement actually contains ingredients in it that can be beneficial. To date, there are no manufacturing standards for herbal supplements. This means there is a wide range of active ingredients in them so the supplements will vary tremendously in their potential effectiveness. Also, because there are no quality control standards, contamination of ingredients and safe use may be a problem.

Although herbal medicine has been around for centuries and has been an effective medical practice globally, it has not been practiced

CHART 1–13

Popular Herbal Supplements

HERB	USE	REPORTED PROBLEMS
Black cohosh	Alleviates PMS	May cause nausea and vomiting
Echinacea	Immune system booster	May stimulate immune system; avoid if you have auto immune problems like lupus or arthritis
Ephedra (Ma Huang)	Weight loss	Dangerous side effects, including high blood pressure, insomnia, anxiety, death
Garlic	Immune system booster, cancer preventer	May cause heartburn or gas
Ginkgo biloba	Memory booster	Check on drug interactions; can raise blood pressure
Green Tea	Memory booster	None reported
St. John's Wort	Antidepressant	Standardization problems; don't use with other antidepressant/anti-anxiety meds
SamE	Antidepressant, osteoarthritis prevention	No long-term studies; can trigger heart problems; don't use if you have obsessive-compulsive disorder

or purchased in the form Americans are enticed into buying today. What we do know about the medicinal benefits of herbal supplements is summarized in Chart 1–13.

What Should You Really Eat?

For years, we have seen the Food Guide Pyramid posted on everything from cereal boxes to menus. Take a second look. It's had a makeover, which means you may need to get reacquainted with it. The "new and improved" Food Guide Pyramid is now called a **Food Guidance System** or MyPyramid (Chart 1–14) and it's sporting a new approach to eating well.

This time around, the new pictorial of healthy eating has a partner—a set of stairs running along the left side of the pyramid. It's there to underscore the importance of activity in staying healthy. The colored

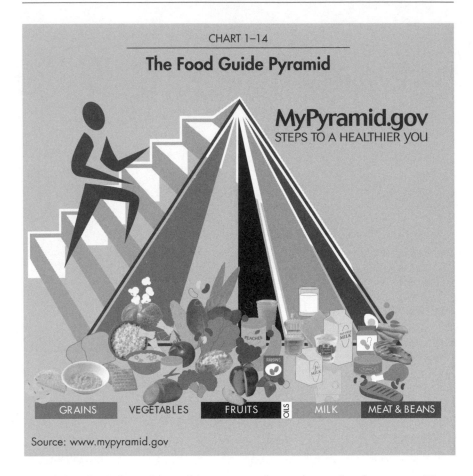

CHART 1–14

The Food Guide Pyramid

MyPyramid.gov
STEPS TO A HEALTHIER YOU

GRAINS   VEGETABLES   FRUITS   OILS   MILK   MEAT & BEANS

Source: www.mypyramid.gov

bands within the pyramid represent the various food groups. They are now vertically placed as compared to the horizontal blocks inside the old pyramid. The new system is a bit more complicated to use, but remains a snapshot of balance, variety, and moderation in eating well.

Recognizing that one diet doesn't fill all . . . MyPyramid is designed to be *your* Pyramid and can be when you log on to www.myPyramid. gov. Once you do, you can use the site to figure out how much food and how many calories you should eat based on your age, gender and level of physical activity. (Chart 1–15) Even with a fairly involved process plugging in information about what and how you eat, the net result is cumbersome and, for many people, difficult to understand. Many who visit the site may still have a tough time answering the question: what and how much should I eat? We'll help answer that question in the next section.

CHART 1-15

Estimated Calorie Range for College-Age Students, Aged 18–22

Females 1800—2400
Males 2200—3000

Daily amount of food from each group for selected calorie ranges

Calorie level	1600	1800	2000	2200	2400	2600	2800
Fruits (cups)	1.5	1.5	2	2	2	2	2.5
Vegetables (cups)	2	2.5	2.5	3	3	3.5	3.5
Grains (oz. equiv)	5	6	6	7	8	9	10
Meat/beans (oz. equiv)	5	5	5.5	6	6.5	6.5	7
Milk (cups)	3	3	3	3	3	3	3
Oils (tsp)	5	5	6	6	7	8	8
Discretionary calories	132	195	267	290	362	410	426

Source: www.mypyramid.gov

MyPyramid . . . Building a Better Diet Block by Block

There are six colored bands in the new pyramid. Each represents a different food group: **grains, vegetables, fruit, dairy, fats** and **protein**. The relative importance of each food group in the diet is shown by the different widths of the bands. The wider the band at the bottom of the pyramid, the greater proportion of your diet it should contain. For example, the orange, green and red bands are wider than the yellow and purple bands, meaning grains, vegetables and fruits should outpace the amount of fat and meats, fish and poultry you eat.

In the original pyramid, the majority of the foods you were encouraged to eat came from the **grains group**. That holds true with the new pyramid as well. This edition of the food pyramid however, makes a distinction between whole grains and refined grains (think oatmeal vs. highly sweetened cereals). The goal is simple and realistic: At least one-half of the grains you eat daily should be whole grains. When you have a choice, choose 100% whole wheat bread, whole grain cereals such as Wheaties and Total and brown rice in place of white rice.

The new pyramid has taken the old amorphous "servings" and put them in what is hoped to be easier to understand portion size terms.

But, it is still difficult to visualize what counts as a one-ounce serving of grains. You can view actual serving sizes at www.mypyramid.gov or take a peek at what counts as a 1 ounce equivalent in Chart 1–16.

The green stripe within the pyramid denotes **vegetables** while the red stripe represents **fruits.** When combined they make up the largest proportion of the diet—more so than grains. MyPyramid categorizes vegetables into five subgroups. This is enough to intimidate any college student who finds it hard to fit those foods into his or her diet to begin with. Don't despair. Look at the portion sizes carefully. Twelve baby carrots could put you half way to your required 2 cups of veggies for the day. As for the five subgroups . . . go for dark green and dark orange when possible and enjoy these crisp, crunchy, colorful foods as often as you like.

When it comes to fruits, servings are now given as cups, with most college students needing about 2 cups each and every day. Nature has neatly packaged most fruit in ready to eat serving sizes, but in the new pyramid, some fruit servings are categorized as a cup, or ½ cup portions. Note that a box of fruit juice can meet the requirement for half of your fruit requirement for a day. To get more fiber and fewer calories, you are encouraged to eat fruit rather than drink fruit juice. To simplify fruit and veggie recommendations, strive to have half of your plate filled with fruits and veggies. You'll be sure to meet the serving guidelines that way.

Perhaps the biggest change coming from the new pyramid is the suggested increase in **dairy** consumption. Two or three servings a day will meet the recommended guidelines for most college students. (If you can't tolerate dairy, be sure to read about substitutions in Chapter 10.)

Serving sizes are given in terms of cups. Milk and yogurt are pretty easy to figure out. A carton of yogurt (ideally lower fat, lower sugared yogurt) is a serving and an 8-ounce box drink of milk is a serving. When it comes to cheese, a 1-ounce slice or 1-inch cube or 3 tablespoons of shredded cheese all equal one serving. Keep in mind cheese is a fairly high fat food (see following discussion on discretionary calories). Its calories can add up quickly.

Protein foods, such as meat, fish, poultry and non-animal sources, are represented by the purple band. Recommendations are given in ounce equivalents. To make the best choices think baked, broiled, boiled, grilled for most of your meals rather than fried and breaded. Since we don't normally weigh our foods, using common ounce equivalents given in Chart 1–16 will make serving recommendation more user friendly.

The thin yellow stripe in the pyramid guides you in choosing the small, but important, **fats** in your diet. The message here: stick with "good" oils (those liquid at room temperature), avoid trans fat (often found in processed foods and labeled as "partially hydrogenated" oils), and don't eat too much of any one kind. Simply put you can use salad dressing, but make it olive or canola oil-based dressings and don't drown the salad.

What about everything else? MyPyramid introduces a brand-new term, "discretionary calories," to account for food choices which may contain more sugar, more fat or fewer nutrients than supplied by the foods we've just talked about. Puddings, ice cream and frozen yogurt are technically in the milk group because of their milk based ingredients, but they most likely take up some of your "discretionary calories" too because of the fair amount of fat and/or sugar they contain. If your protein choices are pre-breaded nuggets (which tend to be high in fat) then they also take up some of your discretionary calories in addition to the protein servings they meet.

Everyone has room for discretionary food choices, but the amounts vary depending on your calorie needs. For many people, the bulk of discretionary calories often come from the foods chosen for taste not nutrition. (Though I'd argue that some of the best tasting foods are also the best for you, such as fresh picked strawberries, a steamy bowl of lentil soup, or a cold glass of skim milk.) Even a healthy diet can contain chips, candy and cookies, but the idea here is to fill up first on the good stuff, then, if interested, include "discretionary" types of foods.

Some foods may seem hard to place within the pyramid. For example, pizza, burritos and sushi fit into more than one category. They can provide you with nutrients from the grain, protein and vegetable groups, so they can be counted as servings from all three. Don't get hung up on a "perfect fit" for all your foods. A healthy diet is a balance of nutritious foods eaten over the course of time. Eating foods from all

CHART 1–16

Portion Equivalents

PYRAMID FOOD GROUP/ SERVING SIZE	WHAT COUNTS AS A SERVING	SIZE COMPARISON
Fruit	**1 cup**	
Apple	½ large apple	
Banana	1	
Grapes	32	
Orange	1	
Strawberries	8	
Raisins	2 small boxes	
Fruit juice	1 cup	
Vegetables	**1 cup**	
Broccoli	3 spears	
Leafy greens, raw	2 cups	
Carrots	12 baby	
Sweet potato	1	Tennis ball
White potato	1	Computer mouse
Tomato juice	1 cup	
Grains	**Ounce equivalents (oz.eq)**	
Bagel	1 bagel counts as 4 oz.eq.	
Bread	1 slice	
Crackers	5–7	
English muffin	½	
Oatmeal	1 packet	
Popcorn	3 cups popped	
1 microwave bag	4 oz. eq.	
Ready to eat cereal	1 cup flakes	1 handful
Pasta	1 cup cooked	Baseball
Tortilla	1 large counts as 4 oz. eq.	
Meat/beans	**Ounce equivalents (oz.eq)**	
Beef/Fish steak	1 serving = 3–4 oz. eq.	Deck of cards
Chicken breast	3–4 oz. eq.	Palm of hand
1 can of tuna, drained	3–4 oz. eq.	
1 egg	1 oz. eq.	
12 almonds	1 oz. eq.	

1 cup bean soup	2 oz. eq.
1 vegetarian burger	2 oz. eq.
2 Tbs. Hummus	1 oz. eq.
1 Tbs. Peanut butter	1 oz. eq.
Dairy	**1 cup**
Skim milk	1 cup or 1 small box drink
Yogurt, 1 container	6–8 oz. container
Cheese, 1–1.5 oz.	⅓ cup shredded
	2 cups cottage cheese
Oils	**Teaspoons**
Vegetable oils	1 Tbs. = 3 tsp.
Mayonnaise	
Salad dressing	1 ladle = 6 tsp.

groups in the pyramid in the proportions recommended, gives you the balance and fuel your body needs. (see Chart 1–17)

Healthy eating means giving your body a variety of foods throughout the day, the week, and the year. Balance is imperative; some meals will be better than others, so will some weeks. Establish a few goals for how you want to eat; remember, how you eat equates, to a large extent, to how you feel.

You neither need a Ph.D. in nutrition to survive and thrive, nor do you probably want one. You do, however, need some food facts, some planning, and an interest in being the best you can be. When you feel good, you look good. When you feel good, life is good.

CHART 1–17

Typical Diets

FOOD GUIDE PYRAMID SERVINGS

THE RESTRICTOR

Breakfast
Cereal bar	1 grain
Orange juice	1 cup fruit

Lunch
8 pieces of vegetable sushi	1 vegetable, 1 grain

Snack
1 Skim latte	1 cup milk

Dinner
Large salad with grilled chicken	1 vegetable, 3 protein equivalents
Diet coke	

Snack
½ bag of microwave popcorn	2.5 grains

This diet is seriously low in calories and major nutrients.
To improve this diet:
    Add at least two servings of whole grains by adding
       a whole wheat roll at dinner
    Add 2 cups of milk by having yogurt at breakfast and milk at dinner
    Add a piece of fruit at lunch
    Add a cup of cooked vegetables at dinner
    Add a tablespoon of olive oil to salad

THE SENSIBLE EATER

Breakfast
1 Packet of oatmeal	2 whole grains, 2 oil
1 Slice whole wheat toast with butter	
Orange juice	1 fruit

Lunch
Peanut butter and jelly sandwich	2 whole grains, 1 protein equivalents, discretionary calories
Skim milk	1 milk
Small bag of chips	discretionary calories
1 apple	2 fruit

Snack
Vegetable soup	2 vegetables

Dinner

Grilled chicken breast	4 protein equivalents
Broccoli	1 vegetable
Rice	1 grain
Salad with oil and vinegar	1 vegetable, 1 oil
Frozen yogurt	discretionary

Snack

1 cup of whole grain cereal	1 whole grain
1 cup of skim milk	1 milk

This diet would meet the pyramid guidelines for someone hoping to come in around 1800 calories. These foods are readily available on college campuses. The key to this diet is portion sizes and limiting in between grazing

EATING WHAT'S EASY

Breakfast

Bagel	4 grains
Coffee	

Lunch

Turkey sub	4 oz. protein equivalent, 4 grains
Bag of chips	discretionary
Soft drink	discretionary

Snack

1 slice of pizza	about 2 grains, 1 dairy, ½ vegetable, and discretionary
Soft drink	discretionary

Dinner

Pasta with tomato sauce	3–4 grains 1 vegetable
Large salad with dressing	1 vegetable, 2 oil
Garlic bread	3 grains with 1 oil
Large glass of milk	1.5 dairy

This diet is presently very top heavy from refined grains. It could come in around 2200 calories and be improved nutritionally with the following changes:

   Order the turkey on whole wheat bread
   Eliminate garlic bread at dinner and get steamed vegetables
   Add slice of cheese to bagel in the morning
   Eliminate one/both of soft drinks
   Add fruit to either breakfast, lunch or dinner

FOR MORE INFORMATION . . .

Books

Duyff, R. 2002. *The American Dietetic Association's Complete Food & Nutrition Guide,* Second Edition. New York: John Wiley.

Willett, W. 2001. *Eat, Drink and Be Healthy: The Harvard Medical School Guide to Healthy Eating.* New York: Simon & Schuster.

Newsletters

Tufts University Diet and Nutrition Letter
www.healthletter.tufts.edu

The University of California at Berkeley Wellness Letter
www.berkeleywellness.com

Nutrition Action Health Letter
www.cspinet.com

Harvard Women's Health Watch
www.harvard.edu/women

Harvard Health Letter
www.health.harvard.edu

Mayo Clinic Health Letter
www.mayohealth.org

2

Eating Well On Campus

You name it, they've got it. Campus eating is a free-for-all; college food services offer a limitless selection of things to eat. The good news is the abundance of healthy choices in the mix. The challenge is to navigate through to them.

Before you maneuver your way through college menus, it helps to come up with a general plan of when you'll eat. Remember that every day your schedule may be different, so the operative word is "general." Can you get what your body needs in just one meal, or is it better to graze, eating throughout the day? How about those late night pizza deliveries—are they a nutritional bonus or a bust?

Starting at the top of the day, breakfast is best. It's the gold medal as far as good health goes. Though it may be tempting to sleep right through the morning meal, skipping breakfast:

- Shortchanges your body, your brain, and your attitude;
- Can make you feel crabby come mid-morning;
- Tends to more than make up for the calories you missed in the morning by overeating in the afternoon and evening.

People who miss breakfast miss out on giving their bodies enough calcium (important for bones), enough folic acid (important for your immune system and energy level), and enough vitamin C (important for keeping your gums and skin healthy).

Breakfast doesn't need to be a big production. The standard offerings, such as cold and hot cereals, baked goods, yogurt, hot entrees, and beverages are great (see Chart 2–1). If you sleep in and wake up midday, consider the first meal you eat as **breaking the fast**. To get your body going, try and eat your meal within an hour of waking. Be creative; breakfast does not need to be breakfast foods.

Make time for lunch **and** dinner, too. If too much time elapses between meals, when you finally sit down to eat, you may feel out of control and overeat. Actually sitting down to eat is more important than a grab-and-go lifestyle. Can you spare five minutes to eat a sandwich? Make the time. It will taste better and you'll probably digest it more smoothly, too.

Under normal conditions it's a good idea to eat every three to four hours; under "college conditions," the same holds true. Because your day often starts late and ends late, a well-rounded snack will help you make it through to the late evening. Although you might have heard that late-night eating is more likely to put on weight, you're not living a 9-to-5 lifestyle. Your eating needs to be adjusted to your college schedule.

Unfortunately, in the wee hours of the morning you are often at the mercy of 24-hour carryout food or, worse, vending machine cuisine. Instead of letting the midnight munchies sneak up on you, plan your day with a late-night meal in mind. Think meal foods rather than

CHART 2–1

Break the Fast

Don't have time for breakfast? These healthy choices can be prepared in three minutes or less . . . with staples found even in a dorm room. Heartier appetites should increase serving size.

	CALORIES	PROTEIN (gm)	FAT (gm)	CHO	FIBER (gm)
Bakery bagel with 1 Tbsp. lite cream cheese or peanut butter Small orange juice	445	15	5	85	.3
1 oz. cereal with skim milk Banana	290	15	1	59	4
English muffin 1 oz. melted mozzarella cheese or ¼ cup cottage cheese Small orange juice	375	11	16	53	2
Hard-boiled egg Toast with margarine Apple sauce	245	9	12	26	4
Instant oatmeal 8 oz. skim milk Small box of raisins	320	14	3	64	4
2 Cereal bars 8 oz. skim milk	290	9	9	46	4
Low-fat yogurt Apple	290	12	3	61	4

snack-type foods such as chips, pretzels, or even rice cakes. In other words, that pizza delivery doesn't have to be your downfall, as long as you've factored in a slice or two as a meal.

Most students have access to a refrigerator, so it's possible to keep some good choices on hand; cereal and milk, soup, and yogurt are great. This late-night eating should be more like a meal, with a beginning and an end, rather than an endless eating orgy (see Chart 2–2).

CHART 2-2				
Satisfying Snack Foods				
	CALORIES	PROTEIN (gm)	FAT (gm)	CHO (gm)
Soup, canned or instant	100	4	2	18
Low-fat yogurt	190	9	3	31
Honey Nut Cheerios and milk	155	6	1.5	28
Instant oatmeal	140	6	2.5	24
Personal pizza*	200	12	4	29
Frozen banana*	100	—	—	25
Granola bar and milk	200	11	4	30

*Recipe in Chapter 14.

That Was When, This Is How

A variety of eating situations is available in college. They more closely resemble a restaurant experience than the home-cooked meals you are used to. The downside to dining in the cafeteria, food court, or group-home such as fraternities and sororities, is the amount of food that is available and served. There are always tempting food choices, portions are usually pretty large, and the food is often prepared with a fair amount of fat. Become a savvy restaurant consumer rather than a cafeteria victim (see Chart 2-3).

Foods that never appeared on your kitchen table at home are now front and center. For example, breakfast at home was toast or cereal; now you have five entrée choices such as waffles and sausage; omelets; or biscuits, bacon, and gravy. A cookie after lunch used to be your mainstay dessert; now you can say hello to soft-serve ice cream, build-your-own sundaes, pies, or cakes. And dinner? It's a smorgasbord of possibilities, each choice more appealing than the next.

How do you select healthy meals from all of the above? It's not a problem with a little planning.

CHART 2–3

Eating Right When Eating Out

If your dining out experience is once in a while, go for it. Eat whatever you want, since an occasional disregard for good nutrition is good for the soul. However, if you find yourself in a restaurant often, which is how many college campus food services operate, have a plan and stick to it.

1. Avoid going into a restaurant ravenously hungry. Everything looks good, and you will no doubt over order and overeat. Instead, eat a piece of fruit or raw vegetables before dining.
2. If you plan on having alcohol, first drink something thirst-quenching, such as water, seltzer, or mineral water. This is especially important if salty snacks and chips are offered before the meal.
3. Restaurant portions tend to be huge. Entrees can be 8-12 ounces instead of the standard portion of 3-6 ounces. Split meals, order appetizer portions, or take a doggie bag to keep your portions in check.
4. Always request toast "dry," "hold the mayo," and sauces and dressings served on the side. If you choose to use them, apply with the tines of the fork or dip the fork in the dressing/sauce, then add the food.
5. Grilled and broiled foods are often brushed with oil before serving. Request that your foods be "grilled dry."
6. Watch out for the "extras" on the table. If the bread basket is a problem, have it removed or placed out of your reach.
7. Fresh fruit is usually available, but not always on the menu.
8. Stop eating before you feel full. Chew slowly, savor each bite, and have uneaten food removed promptly.
9. Have your water glass refilled during the meal.
10. If you're ordering many dishes to share, as you might do in a Chinese restaurant, put all of your choices on the plate before you begin. Then, stop after one plate. Don't keep adding small amounts; they add up quickly.

Manage the Menu

The all-you-can-eat concept in most college food services is an open invitation to overeat. Three simple steps can help you manage the menu:

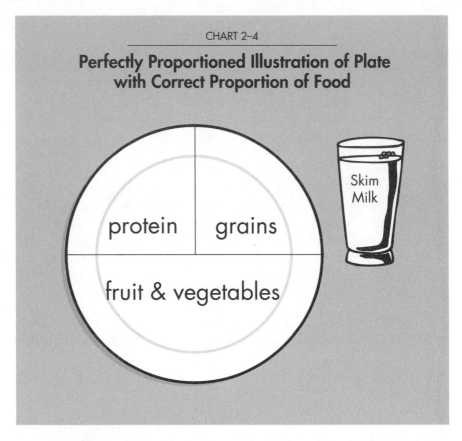

CHART 2–4

**Perfectly Proportioned Illustration of Plate
with Correct Proportion of Food**

- Walk through the whole line to get the lay of the land—in other words, see what's for dinner.
- Decide on what looks good. Fruit and/or vegetables should be front and center (see Chart 2–4). Put all you need on the plate, and don't go back for seconds.
- A **very** hungry person makes poor choices, so try not to arrive at meals famished . . . or at least be aware of your impulsive need to eat anything and everything and proceed with care.

More Specifics: Cafeteria Menu

Most cafeterias offer a combination of self-serve or served tray lines. You can keep that healthy spirit alive as you wind your way through some of the offerings. Here's how:

CHART 2–5

Super Salad Bars

- Start with leafy greens like lettuce and spinach.
- Pile high other fresh veggies, like carrots, mushrooms, cucumbers, peppers.
- Limit the prepared salads, such as pasta salad, marinated vegetable salad, and potato salad.
- Choose "plain protein" choices like cottage cheese, eggs, tuna, cheese, chickpeas, tofu, and turkey to make your salad an entrée rather than a side.
- Skip the extras like croutons, bacon bits, fried noodles.
- Dress the salad first with vinegar, salsa, or lemon; then add a limited amount of olive oil or dressing of your choice.

	SERVING SIZE	CALORIES	FAT	PROTEIN	CHO
Veggies					
Artichoke hearts	¼ cup	18	0	1	3.5
Bean sprouts	¼ cup	8	0	1	1
Beets	¼ cup	20	0	0.5	4
Broccoli	½ cup	12	0	1	2.5
Cabbage	½ cup	8	0	0.5	1.5
Carrots, shredded	¼ cup	15	0	0	4
Cauliflower	½ cup	12	0	0	2.5
Celery	¼ cup	5	0	0	1.5
Corn	¼ cup	33	0.5	2	8
Cucumbers	¼ cup	4	0	0	1
Hearts of palm	¼ cup	10	0	1	1
Lettuce	1 cup	12	0	0	2
Mushrooms	¼ cup	9	0	1	1
Onions	1 Tbsp.	4	0	0	1
Peas	2 Tbsp.	30	0	2	5
Peppers, red or green	2 Tbsp.	7	0	0	1
Radishes	¼ cup	6	0	0	1
Spinach	1 cup	7		1	1
Squash, yellow or green	¼ cup			0	1
Tomatoes, chopped	½ cup			1	3
Protein Choices					
Cheese, cottage (creamed)	½ cup	120	5	14	6
Cheese, cottage (low-fat)	½ cup	80	2	12	3
Cheese, shredded cheddar	3 Tbsp.	115	10	7	—

	SERVING SIZE	CALORIES	FAT	PROTEIN	CHO
Cheese, grated Parmesan	2 Tbsp.	45	3	4	—
Chickpeas	½ cup	140	2	6	27
Eggs, chopped	2 Tbsp.	25	2	7	0
Tofu	½ cup	94	6	10	4
Turkey, diced	2 Tbsp.	50	1.5	10	0
Tuna, plain	2 Tbsp.	60	1	13	0

Prepared Salads

	SERVING SIZE	CALORIES	FAT	PROTEIN	CHO
Carrot raisin	¼ cup	130	5	1	22
Macaroni	½ cup	135	5	3	21
Marinated artichoke	¼ cup	41	3	1	3
Pasta	½ cup	150	8	2.5	16
Potato	½ cup	179	10	3	14
Three-bean	½ cup	70	4	2	7
Tuna	¼ cup	96	5	8	5
Waldorf (apples, nuts)	½ cup	96	6	1	10

Extras

	SERVING SIZE	CALORIES	FAT	PROTEIN	CHO
Bacon bits	1 Tbsp.	25	1	1	5
Chow mein noodles	½ cup	115	7	2	13
Croutons	2 Tbsp.	50	2	1	6
Olives	5	25	2	0	0
Pickles	1	5	0	0	1
Raisins	1 Tbsp.	60	0	0	13
Sunflower seeds	2 Tbsp.	180	16	7	9

Dressings*

	SERVING SIZE	CALORIES	FAT	PROTEIN	CHO
Bleu cheese	2 Tbsp.	160	16	1	2
Bleu cheese, fat-free	2 Tbsp.	36	0	0	7
Caesar	2 Tbsp.	158	18	1	1
Caesar, fat-free	2 Tbsp.	30	0	0	7
French	2 Tbsp.	120	11	0	5
French, fat-free	2 Tbsp.	43	1	0	8
Italian	2 Tbsp.	140	15	0	3
Ranch	2 Tbsp.	180	20	0	1
Ranch, fat-free	2 Tbsp.	34	0	0	7
Salsa	2 Tbsp.	8	0	0	2
Soy sauce	2 Tbsp.	10	0	1	2
Thousand Island	2 Tbsp.	160	15	0	9
Thousand Island, fat-free	2 Tbsp.	50	0	0	10
Vinegar	2 Tbsp.	4	0	0	1
Vinegarette	2 Tbsp.	60	5	0	3

*1 "ladle" of dressing at a salad bar = 4 Tbsp.

Salad Bars

It's a sink-or-swim situation at the salad bar. Eating fresh vegetables is certainly nutrition nirvana. However, some salad bar items are not exactly "harvested from the soil." Many are loaded with mayonnaise, salad dressing, or even whipped cream (see Chart 2–5).

Baked Potato Bars

Baked potato bars are a popular spot where an entire meal can revolve around a solitary spud. Pile veggies on your potato and a little au jus (broth), and you have a real meal (see Chart 2–6).

CHART 2–6

Building a Better Baked Potato

	CALORIES	PROTEIN (gm)	CHO (gm)	FAT (gm)
Plain	212	5	49	0
Broccoli and cheddar	139	12.5	12	9
Spinach and cottage cheese	108	17	8	1
Steamed veggies and Parmesan cheese	71	6.5	5.5	4
Stir-fried and tofu	215	10	7	17.5
Marinara sauce and Parmesan cheese	154	6	18	6
Salsa and cheddar	134	10	11	9
Plain yogurt	75	6	9	1.5
Chili	145	8	9	3

Sandwiches

Sandwiches remain the cornerstone of most lunches. Two slices of crusty, whole grain bread become terrific companions for a variety of protein choices such as turkey, ham, or peanut butter. Pitas, English muffins, small rolls, and the currently popular wraps are great to make sandwiches, too. If you're trying to avoid extra calories, stay away from large sub rolls, croissants, bakery-size bagels, and paninis. Pass by the overstuffed sandwiches, fries, and shakes. Instead, round out your sandwich by adding fruit, broth-based soup, or a crunchy veggie salad. Substitute mustard, barbecue sauce, or salsa for mayonnaise or adorn your meat choice with sprouts, tomatoes, or cucumbers, and you'll have pretty healthy fare (see Chart 2–7).

CHART 2–7

Stacking Up Your Favorite Sandwiches

	CALORIES	FAT (gm)	PROTEIN (gm)	CHO (gm)
Turkey on whole wheat	260	4	27	30
Roast beef on rye	310	7	31	32
Tuna on pita*	340	5	37	78
Grilled cheese	310	18	10	25
PB & J	350	10	10	60
Grilled chicken sandwich	280	3	29	30
Tuna sub (12 in)	900	92	40	44
Steak & cheese sub (12 in)	780	96	40	26
Meatball sub (6 in)	530	26	24	53
Slice of pizza	250	10	12	28
Chicken Caesar wrap	460	11	38	51
Turkey panini	670	23	47	68

* Tuna packed in oil.

Hot Entrées

Entrées run the gamut from tofu pie to fried chicken (see Chart 2–8). A healthy sounding entrée can still pile on fat and calories though. Many colleges employ qualified nutritionists who can answer specific questions about the foods being served. Ask questions about how foods are prepared; make requests, such as serving sauces on the side; and be a menu sleuth by uncovering the real meaning behind how foods are advertised (see Chart 2–9). If nothing looks appealing, stick to the basics—salad, bread, veggies, pasta, or cereal. A bowl of cereal and milk is a perfectly acceptable dinner when all else fails.

CHART 2–8

Lunch and Dinner Ideas that Pass the Cafeteria Test

Entrées

Sandwiches made on bread, pita, tortilla, small roll, or bagel

Turkey, roast beef, ham and cheese, grilled chicken, peanut butter and jelly, or tuna*

Plain, veggie, and turkey burgers

Cheese or veggie pizza

Grilled or broiled chicken (skinless)

Grilled or broiled fish

Lean meat strips

Bean soups

Vegetarian chili

Fajitas

Building a better baked potato (See Chart 2–6)

Super salad bars (See Chart 2-5)

*Request water-packed Tuna

Plain pasta with tomato sauce

Scrambled, poached, or hard-boiled eggs

Plain rice and steamed vegetables

Sides

Broth-based or tomato-based soups

Steamed or fresh vegetables

Fresh fruit

Canned fruit

Plain breads, rolls, bagels

Baked potato

Corn on the cob

Steamed rice

Skim, low-fat milk, or soy milk

Yogurt

CHART 2-9

Deciphering the Language of Menus

The guidelines listed here should help you to navigate even the standard cafeteria menu.

This is a better choice . . .	Than this
Roasted	Au gratin or cheese sauce
Steamed	Fried
Marinara sauce	Alfredo
Grilled	Scampi style
Cooked in its own juice	Cooked with butter, cream
Barbecued	Batter-dipped, tempura
Broiled	Breaded
Poached	Sautéed
Tomato sauce	Cream sauce, gravy

Desserts

Desserts offer something tasty at the end of the meal. Healthy sounding or not, desserts are essentially extra calories. Fat-free delicacies, frozen yogurt, or fruit pies may sound healthier, but they're still desserts (calories, but not much nutrition). If calories are a concern, keep your dessert pick to either lunch **or** dinner, or maybe limit your desserts to one or two days a week. If you have unlimited access to the frozen yogurt machine, try putting it on a cone rather than in a cup, or you may be better off not starting at all. Find a friend and share a dessert. Or better yet, recall that motherly suggestion, "Why not have a piece of fruit for dessert, dear?" (see Chart 2–10).

CHART 2–10

Delicious Desserts

Desserts are a part of a healthy diet, but not every meal needs to end with one. Choose the large, gooey ones occasionally and the others listed below more often.

Fresh fruit	Skim milk latte or cappuccino
Frozen desserts	3 small or 1 large cookie
Fruit bars	Baked apple
Yogurt bars	Applesauce
Popsicles	
Fudgesicles	
Ice Cream sandwiches	
Low-fat ice cream, ice milk, or	
frozen yogurt	
Sorbet	

Fast Food Menus

Fast food is part of life, and it's certainly part of college life. How much fast food can you eat and still be healthy? It's hard to say. Even though fast food menus have expanded beyond burgers, fries, and shakes, the choices are limited, particularly when it comes to fruits and vegetables. Variety and moderation are key to eating well, so fast food can fit in, but it cannot have exclusive rights to your meal plans.

Pay attention to portions. "Super size," "value meals," and "over-stuffed" translate into overindulgence. Stick with regular-size servings. If a small burger doesn't fill you up, make a second choice only after you have finished eating your first round of food. Plain burgers and sandwiches are better selections because extra sauces, cheese, and dressings add fat, salt, and calories. Breaded chicken and fish sandwiches often have more fat and calories than plain burgers. Don't be fooled by salads either. They may sound healthy, but the more stuff on them, the more stuff in them (as in calories and fat) (see Chart 2–11).

Group-Home Menus

Eating your meals in a small-group setting, such as a sorority or fraternity house, may pose a whole new set of circumstances. The food choices are more limited at group homes, but because the number of people being served is smaller, you may actually be able to influence what is prepared. If you sit down to your first few meals and they're not what you were hoping for, be proactive. See if you can connect with the cook. Maybe you can form a committee to help plan menus. Poll your housemates and get together a list of seven to ten meals everyone likes. If the cook isn't familiar with healthy cooking techniques, provide him or her with resources and recipes.

Other Tips

Make no mistake; eating is a social event. At home you may have wanted to dine and dash, but now meals are a great time to hang out with friends. The problem is that you are essentially sitting in a sea of food—it's all around you and it's hard to resist. To avoid overeating:

- Sit far away from where food is served.
- Promptly remove your tray and anything you haven't eaten as soon as you are full. If uneaten food stares at you long enough, you start nibbling—avoid the urge.

- If you plan to stock up for late-night snacks, fill your pockets with foods that are packed with nutrition, not just calories. Select fruit or mini boxes of cereal, not rolls, cookies, or donuts which taste good going down, but are not so good once they get there.
- Pay attention to your food while you're eating, then socialize. This way you can focus on how much you've eaten.

Try varying where you eat so that you can vary your food choices, too. For instance, have breakfast in your room, lunch at the fast food restaurant on campus, and dinner in a traditional cafeteria. A healthy diet is a balance of different kinds of foods that offer different kinds of nutrients. Three meals a day from a limited menu won't give you the balance you need.

Food service providers, whether they're in a group living situation or in a dorm, are hired to meet the needs of their customers. If you don't see what you like, ask for it. Innovations ranging from 24-hour service to "made to order" are the result of consumer feedback.

A complete nutrient analysis is often available for everything on the cafeteria line or fast food menu. Plan when, where, and how you want to eat, and open your mind to trying new foods. Do it and you will graduate not only with a college degree, but with a healthy body as well.

CHART 2–11

Fast Food Follies

	CALORIES	CHO (gm)	PROTEIN (gm)	FAT (gm)
Bruegger's Bagels				
Plain bagel	300	61	12	2
Poppy bagel	310	61	12	3
Garlic	310	61	12	2
Cinnamon raisin	320	68	11	2
Sesame	320	61	12	2
Plain Cream Cheese (2 Tbsp.)	90	4	2	8
Plain Light Cream Cheese (2 Tbsp.)	70	3	2	5
Dunkin' Donuts				
Bagels				
Plain bagel	320	62	12	3
Poppyseed	370	65	14	7
Cinnamon raisin	330	65	10	3
Sesame	380	64	14	8
Donuts				
Old-fashioned	300	28	4	19
Glazed	180	25	3	8
Powdered	330	36	4	19
Chocolate Kreme filled	270	35	3	13
Munchkins				
Glazed (5)	200	27	3	9
Glazed Chocolate (3)	200	26	2	10
Sugar Raised (7)	220	26	4	12
Powdered (4)	270	31	3	14
Plain croissant	330	37	5	18
Muffins				
Blueberry	470	73	8	17
Blueberry, reduced fat	440	75	8	12
Chocolate Chip	630	89	10	26
Banana Walnut	540	73	10	23
English muffin	160	32	6	2
Coolatta				
Coffee Coolatta® with Milk	210	42	4	4
Coffee Coolatta® with Skim Milk	170	41	4	0
Strawberry Fruit Coolatta®	290	72	0	0

	CALORIES	CHO (gm)	PROTEIN (gm)	FAT (gm)
Krispy Kreme Doughnuts				
Original glazed	200	22	2	12
Chocolate iced	250	33	3	12
Glazed raspberry filled	300	39	3	16
Glazed cruller	240	26	2	14
Chocolate iced with sprinkles	260	38	3	12
Cinnamon bun	260	28	3	16
Traditional cake	230	25	3	13
Powdered cake	280	37	3	14
Arby's				
Sandwiches				
Market Fresh Low Carbys				
Roast Ham & Swiss	200	5	26	9
Market Fresh Low Carbys Ultimate BLT	210	6	13	17
Italian Beef 'n Provolone	650	54	40	31
Philly Beef Supreme	730	56	36	40
Market Fresh Low Carbys Wrap				
Roast Turkey Ranch & Bacon	710	50	48	40
Market Fresh Low Carbys Wrap				
Ultimate BLT	660	50	24	47
Chicken Breast Fillet	540	47	24	30
Grilled Chicken Deluxe	410	39	29	16
Salads				
Martha's Vineyard Salad	280	22	26	10
Santa Fe Salad	520	40	27	29
Santa Fe Ranch Dressing	264	3	1	28
Asian Sesame Salad	170	14	21	3
Asian Sesame Dressing	190	15	1	14
Light Buttermilk Ranch Dressing	100	12	1	6
Light Vinaigrette	110	13	0	6
Fat Free Italian	30	7	0	0
Turkey Club Salad (No dressing)	350	9	33	21
Caesar Salad	90	8	7	4
Grilled Chicken Caesar	230	8	33	8
Chicken Finger Salad	570	39	30	34
Other				
Curly Fries™	310	39	4	15
Broccoli 'N Cheddar Baked Potato	540	71	12	24
Jalapeno Bites™	350	30	7	21

	CALORIES	CHO (gm)	PROTEIN (gm)	FAT (gm)
Baja Fresh				
Burritos				
Baja Burrito, steak	890	70	59	42
Baja Burrito, chicken	800	70	54	34
Burrito Mexicano, steak	900	119	56	20
Burrito Mexicano, chicken	810	119	51	13
Burrito Ultimo, steak	990	87	60	42
Burrito Ultimo, chicken	890	87	56	35
Vegetarian Burrito	810	96	33	32
Veggie Bare Burrito	590	102	20	10
Tacos and Taquitos				
Taco Chilito, steak	340	38	21	12
Taco Chilito, chicken	320	38	20	10
Taquitos, steak with rice	790	67	32	42
Taquitos, steak with beans	820	69	40	42
Taquitos, chicken with rice	710	64	30	36
Taquitos, chicken with beans	820	69	40	42
Fajitas				
Fajitas, steak with corn tortilla	1020	116	70	30
Fajitas, steak with flour tortilla	1190	133	76	38
Fajitas, chicken with corn tortilla	870	116	62	19
Fajitas, chicken with flour tortilla	1050	133	75	29
Quesadillas and nachos				
Quesadilla, steak	1350	80	81	79
Quesadilla, chicken	1260	80	76	71
Quesadilla, cheese	1110	75	48	69
Nachos, cheese	1880	166	65	103
Nachos, steak	2100	166	98	113
Salads and soup				
Baja Ensalada, steak	450	18	54	18
Baja Ensalada, chicken	310	18	46	7
Baja ensalada, Shrimp	180	17	21	4
Chile Lime chicken salad	640	75	51	16
With dressing	810	80	51	32
Chipotle glazed chicken salad	600	56	47	22
With dressing	770	64	47	31
Tortilla soup	220	21	7	12
Tostada, steak	1230	100	66	60
Tostada, chicken	1140	100	61	52
Tostada, vegetarian	1010	100	32	50
Side Orders				
Rice	280	55	0.5	4
Black beans	360	61	23	2.5
Pinto beans	320	56	19	1
Guacamole, 3 oz. side	110	7	2	9

	CALORIES	CHO (gm)	PROTEIN (gm)	FAT (gm)
Burger King				
Burgers				
Whopper	760	52	35	46
Whopper with Cheese	850	53	39	53
Double Whopper	1060	52	59	69
Whopper Jr.	390	32	17	22
Hamburger	310	31	17	13
Cheeseburger	360	31	19	17
Bacon Cheeseburger	400	31	22	20
Sandwiches				
BK Fish	710	66	24	39
Chicken Whopper	580	48	39	26
Veggie Burger	330	45	14	10
Grilled Chicken Caesar Club	540	40	34	27
Chicken Tenders				
Chicken Tenders, 4 pc.	170	10	11	9
Chicken Tenders, 6 pc.	250	15	16	14
Fries				
Small Fries	230	29	3	11
Large Fries	500	63	6	25
Chick-fil-A'				
Chicken Sandwich	410	38	28	16
Chargrilled chicken sandwich	280	30	26	7
Chargrilled chicken club sandwich	370	31	32	13
Chick-n-Strips®	290	14	29	13
Nuggets	260	12	26	12
Chicken salad sandwich	350	32	20	15
Hearty Breast of Chicken Soup (reg.)	140	18	8	3.5
Chargrilled chicken garden salad	180	9	22	6
Chicken-n-Strips salad	390	22	34	18
Polynesian Sauce	110	13	0	6
Dijon Honey Mustard Sauce	50	2	0	5
Chipotle				
13" Flour tortilla	330	54	9	9
Crispy taco shell (4 ea.)	240	34	4	9
Rice (5 oz.)	240	40	4	7
Black beans (4 oz.)	130	22	9	1
Pinto beans (4 oz.)	138	23	9	1
Fajita Vegetables (3 oz.)	100	6	1	8
Carnita (4 oz.)	227	0	29	12
Chicken (4 oz.)	219	0	29	11
Steak (4 oz.)	230	2	29	12
Tomato Salsa (4 oz.)	25	6	1	0

	CALORIES	CHO (gm)	PROTEIN (gm)	FAT (gm)
Cheese (1 oz.)	110	<1	7	9
Sour Cream (2 oz.)	120	2	2	10
Guacamole (4 oz.)	170	8	2	15
Lettuce (1 oz.)	5	<1	<1	0
Burrito, rice beans, meat, cheese	1044	117	58	38
Vegetarian burrito, rice, beans				
Sour cream, guacamole	986	126	26	42
Fajita burrito: rice, veggies,				
Meat, salsa	924	106	44	36
Fajita burrito bol: rice, veggies,	674	46	41	36
Meat, cheese				
Bol salad, beans, guacamole	420	52	15	17
Bol salad, veggies, meat, salsa	356	13	32	20

Cosi

Pizza

	CALORIES	CHO (gm)	PROTEIN (gm)	FAT (gm)
Traditional Cheese	1081	125	49	40
Meatlovers	1315	124	61	60
Four Cheese	981	124	35	35
Spinach and fresh tomato	916	129	30	30

Other

	CALORIES	CHO (gm)	PROTEIN (gm)	FAT (gm)
Spinach Artichoke	182	9	6	15
Brie and Fruit	277	26	9	15
Hummus dip	121	18	3	4

Sandwiches

	CALORIES	CHO (gm)	PROTEIN (gm)	FAT (gm)
Grilled Chicken TBM	670	58	44	29
Tuscan Pesto Chicken	571	58	43	22
Hummus and Fresh Veggies	440	75	16	8
Smoked Turkey and Brie	771	73	43	35
Turkey Light	475	75	31	8
Tuna & cheddar	960	56	58	54

Melts

	CALORIES	CHO (gm)	PROTEIN (gm)	FAT (gm)
Tomato, Basil, Mozarella	626	61	29	29
Pesto Chicken	709	61	50	33
Tuna melt	922	57	58	50

Soups

	CALORIES	CHO (gm)	PROTEIN (gm)	FAT (gm)
Chicken Noodle (cup)	116	11	10	4
Three Bean Chili (cup)	162	34	9	1
Minestrone (cup)	174	28	8	3
Lentil (cup)	199	32	13	3
Grilled Chicken Corn Chowder (cup)	305	24	16	16
New England Clam Chowder (cup)	440	24	22	29

Bread

	CALORIES	CHO (gm)	PROTEIN (gm)	FAT (gm)
Cosi Bread (full slice)	265	49	9	3

	CALORIES	CHO (gm)	PROTEIN (gm)	FAT (gm)
Salads				
Shanghai Chicken	222	16	28	5
Signature	370	39	15	21
Greek	222	10	11	17
Caesar	182	20	8	8
Add chicken	340	21	33	16
Bombay Chicken	176	13	27	3
Salad Dressings				
Lowfat Ginger Soy	80	13	1	3
Roasted Shallot Sherry Vinaigrette	300	6	0	32
Reduced Fat Shallot Sherry	80	12	1	3
Low Carb Shallot	314	1	0	34
Caesar Dressing	345	2	2	37
Fat Free Balsamic Vinaigrette	45	11	0	0
Dessert				
S'mmm . . . oreos (for two)	827	147	12	2
S'mores (for two)	751	133	10	21
Mud Pie	850	109	9	49
Fruit salad	216	54	4	1
Double scoop ice cream	225	22	4	14
Blondie brownie	570	57	6	36
Domino's Pizza				
Barbecue wings (1 piece)	50	1.5	5.5	2
Hot wings (1 piece)	45	0.5	5.5	2
Buffalo Kickers (1 piece)	47	3	4	2
Breadsticks (1 piece)	116	17.5	3	4
Cheesy bread (1 piece)	142	17.5	4.5	6
Hand-tossed pizza (per slice of large)				
Cheese	258	37.5	10.5	7.5
Pepperoni	366	38.5	16.5	17
Meatzza	376	17	39	17.5
Vegi	302	39	13.5	11
Thin crust (per ¼ of large pizza)				
Cheese	382	43.5	17	16.5
Jamba Juice				
Smoothies				
Banana Berry™, sixteen	310	74	3	0.5
Banana Berry™, original	480	112	58	18
Chocolate Moo'd®, sixteen	500	102	12	6
Chocolate Moo'd®, original	720	148	17	8
Coldbuster®, sixteen	290	66	4	1.5
Coldbuster®, original	430	100	5	2.5

	CALORIES	CHO (gm)	PROTEIN (gm)	FAT (gm)
Jamba Powerboost®, sixteen	290	69	5	1
Jamba Powerboost®, original	440	105	6	1.5
Strawberries Wild®, sixteen	290	69	4	0
Strawberries Wild®, original	450	105	6	0.5
Kiwi Berry Burner®, sixteen	310	73	2	0
Kiwi Berry Burner®, original	470	112	4	0.5
McDonald's				
Hamburger	260	33	13	9
Cheeseburger	310	35	15	12
Quarter Pounder	420	38	23	18
Quarter Pounder w/cheese	510	43	29	25
Big Mac	560	46	25	30
Crispy Chicken Sandwich	510	47	22	26
Fillet-O-Fish	410	41	22	26
Chicken McGrill®	400	37	27	16
Small French fries	230	30	2	11
Large French fries	520	70	6	25
Chicken McNuggets (6 piece)	250	15	15	15
Chicken McNuggets (10 piece)	420	26	25	24
Chicken Selects® (5 pieces)	630	46	39	33
Barbecue Sauce (1 pkg.)	45	10	0	0
Chipotle Barbecue Sauce (1 pkg.)	70	16	2	0
Sweet 'N Sour Sauce (1 pkg.)	50	11	0	0
Hot Mustard (1 pkg.)	60	7	<1	3.5
Honey (1 pkg.)	45	12	0	0
Light Mayonnaise (1 pkg.)	45	<1	0	4.5
Grilled Chicken California Cobb	270	9	4	11
Crispy Chicken California Cobb	370	20	27	21
Grilled Chicken Bacon Ranch	250	9	31	10
Crispy Chicken Bacon Ranch	350	20	26	19
Grilled Chicken Caesar	200	9	29	6
Crispy Chicken Caesar	310	20	23	16
Croutons (1 pkg.)	50	8	1	1.5
Newman's Own® Cobb Dressing (1 pkg.)	120	9	1	9
Newman's Own® Creamy Caesar Dressing (1 pkg.)	190	4	2	18
Newman's Own® Low Fat Balsamic Vinaigrette	40	4	0	3
Newman's Own® Ranch Dressing (1 pkg.)	290	4	1	30
Fruit 'n Yogurt Parfait	160	30	4	2

	CALORIES	CHO (gm)	PROTEIN (gm)	FAT (gm)
Noodles & Company				
Salads				
Caesar Salad (5.8 oz.)	306	8	10	26
Caesar Salad with Chicken (9 oz.)	445	8	29	33
Market Salad with Fat Free Asian dressing	155	30	3	2.5
Noodle Bowls				
Japanese Pan Noodles (no oil, 16.6 oz.)	630	132	22	1.5
Roma Tomato Marinara (no Cheese)	488	89	15	8
Thai Curry soup	356	38	6	20
Thai Curry soup, chicken no noodles	395	15	23	27
Panera Bread				
Soups (8oz.)				
Broccoli cheddar	230	13	8	16
Low-fat chicken noodle	100	15	5	2
French Onion	220	23	9	10
Baked Potato	260	23	6	16
Low-fat Vegetarian black bean	160	31	9	1
Low-fat garden vegetable (8 oz.)	90	17	4	0.5
Sandwiches				
Turkey artichoke panini	810	76	41	38
Frontega chicken panini	860	71	49	42
Smokehouse turkey panini	670	68	47	23
Asiago roast beef	730	54	50	35
Tuscan chicken	950	76	35	56
Garden Veggie	570	74	15	23
Smoked turkey on Sourdough	440	44	29	15
Italian Combo	1050	80	60	54
Salads				
Grilled chicken caesar	500	19	31	34
Asian sesame chicken	330	34	32	17
Fandango (9.5 oz.)	400	21	7	28
Greek (14 oz.)	520	17	9	48
Breads				
Sourdough soup bowl	500	102	20	1.5
Ciabatta	430	70	14	10
French Croissant	260	28	5	15
French Roll	140	28	6	1
Pastries and sweets				
Chocolate chipper cookie	420	51	5	22
Cinnamon Roll	560	64	12	26
Very chocolate brownie	460	62	5	22

	CALORIES	CHO (gm)	PROTEIN (gm)	FAT (gm)
PF Chang's (values given for whole dish)				
Main dishes				
Beef Mongolian	1080	18	85	72
Beef with broccoli	760	23	56	49
Beef Lo Mein	850	90	47	34
Almond Cashew Chicken	740	51	62	30
Chang's Spicy Chicken	990	70	61	51
Chicken Chow Mein	828	96	48	28
Kung Pao Chicken	1230	51	81	78
Mu shu Chicken	750	55	63	31
Ginger Chicken and broccoli	620	43	63	21
Soups and starters				
Steamed Vegetable Dumplings	300	47	9	8
Fried Vegetable Dumplings	340	47	9	12
Steamed Shrimp Dumplings	320	26	24	12
Fried Shrimp Dumplings	360	26	24	17
Spring rolls	640	106	15	17
Spare ribs	1090	6	49	95
Hot & Sour Soup (1 serving)	56	2	3	4
Wonton (1 serving)	52	4	3	3
Oriental Chicken Salad	940	49	60	56
Peanut-Lime Chicken Salad	1080	47	73	69
Ahi Tuna (appetizer)	220	18	25	5
Noodles and Rice				
Garlic Noodles	610	107	19	12
Vegetable Fried Rice	820	147	25	12
Fried Rice Combo	1130	150	61	28
Vegetables and vegetarian main dishes				
Vegetable lo mein	550	93	21	12
Buddha Feast steamed	200	44	10	1
Buddha Feast stir-fried	370	64	21	7
Garlic Snap Peas	220	20	6	7
Szechwan Asparagus	170	29	11	4
Stir fried eggplant	510	60	8	29
Quizno's Subs				
Sandwiches				
Honey Bourbon Chicken (small)	300	45	24	6
Sierra Smoked Turkey w/Raspberry Chipotle Sauce (small)	358	53	23	6
Turkey Lite (small)	358	52	24	6
Tuscan Chicken Salad (small)	325	45	21	6.3
Veggie Lite (small)	300	40	20	6

	CALORIES	CHO (gm)	PROTEIN (gm)	FAT (gm)
Ranch 1				
Salads				
Chicken on Gourmet Greens (15.2 oz.)	351	31	32	11
Gourmet Greens (5 oz.)	227	31	10	7
Zesty Caesar Salad (6 oz.)	183	31	8	3
Zesty Chicken Caesar Salad (9.2 oz.)	282	31	26	6
Sandwiches				
American Rancher (9 oz.)	394	51	25	10
Club Sandwich (8.6 oz.)	472	53	29	16
Grilled Chicken Philly (8.8 oz.)	450	53	28	14
Ranch Classic (8.7 oz.)	361	53	26	5
Spicy Grilled Chicken (9 oz.)	423	58	23	11
Sides				
Ranch Fries Large (5.5 oz.)	427	62.2	6.1	17.1
Fruit Cup (8.3 oz.)	89	18	3	.5
Specialties				
Baked Potato with Broccoli (18 oz.)	521	117	12	0.5
Baked Potato with Cheese (27.8 oz.)	789	118	26	25
Baked Potato with Chicken (21.5 oz.)	612	114	30	4
Chicken Tenders (All white meat, 13 oz.)	371	7	52	15
Grilled Chicken Fajita (11.6 oz.)	332	25	22	16
Grilled Chicken Hot Pasta (20.8 oz.)	582	86	37	10
Grilled Chicken & Vegetable Platter (25 oz.)	795	129	54	7
Sbarro Pizza				
Pizza (1 Slice)				
Cheese Pizza	488	55.5	23.6	17.8
Pepperoni Pizza	591	55.5	28.9	26.8
Gourmet Vegetable Pizza	837	85.3	29.5	39.7
Calzone/Stuffed Pizza				
Cheese Calzone	776	84.3	41.5	28.2
Stuffed Pizza, Spinach and Broccoli	825	84.6	32.7	39.5
Pasta				
Baked Ziti	928	90.2	44.2	42.3
Meat Lasagna	824	67.8	41.6	41.2
Spaghetti with Sauce	911	144	26.6	22.8
Southern Tsunami (sushi)				
Sushi				
California Roll (9 pieces)	289	54	7	5
Nigiri, Eel (1 piece)	85	13.4	3	2.2
Nigiri, Octopus (1 piece)	66	12.4	3.4	0.3
Nigiri, Salmon (1 piece)	64	12	2.6	0.6
Avocado Roll (small roll, 12 pieces)	292	51.9	5.4	7

	CALORIES	CHO (gm)	PROTEIN (gm)	FAT (gm)
Cucumber Roll (small roll, 12 pieces)	224	49.9	4.8	0.6
Vegetarian Roll (9 pieces)	232	45	4	4
Tuna Roll (small roll, 12 pieces)	258	47	14	1.5
Rainbow Roll (9 pieces)	514	92	14	10
Tempura Roll (9 pieces)	604	92.6	28.6	13.2
Spicy Salmon Roll (9 pieces)	362	52.4	18.3	8.8
Spicy Tuna Roll (9 pieces)	290	45	14	6

Starbucks

Hot Beverages

Brewed Coffee

Tall	5	1	0	0
Grande	10	2	0	0
Venti	15	3	0	0

Caffe Latte

Tall				
Nonfat Milk	120	18	12	0
Whole Milk	200	16	11	11
Soy US	160	21	8	4–5
Grande				
Nonfat Milk	160	24	16	0
Whole Milk	260	21	14	14
Soy US	210	28	11	6
Venti				
Nonfat Milk	210	30	20	0
Whole Milk	340	27	18	18
Soy US	270	36	14	8

Caffe Mocha (with whipped cream)

Tall				
Nonfat Milk	280	34	11	11
Whole Milk	340	33	10	19
Soy US	300	37	8	15
Grande				
Nonfat Milk	330	44	14	12
Whole Milk	400	42	13	22
Soy US	360	48	10	16
Venti				
Nonfat Milk	390	56	19	12
Whole Milk	490	53	17	26
Soy US	440	60	13	18

Carmel Macchiato

Tall				
Nonfat Milk	130	22	9	0.5
Whole Milk	190	20	8	9
Soy US	160	24	6	4

	CALORIES	CHO (gm)	PROTEIN (gm)	FAT (gm)
Grande				
Nonfat Milk	230	40	14	2
Whole Milk	320	37	12	14
Soy US	300	49	9	8
Venti				
Nonfat Milk	280	46	18	2
Whole Milk	390	43	16	17
Soy US	330	51	12	9
Hot Chocolate (without whipped cream)				
Tall				
Nonfat Milk	190	35	13	1.5
Whole Milk	270	33	12	12
Soy US	230	38	9	6
Grande				
Nonfat Milk	240	45	16	2
Whole Milk	340	42	15	15
Soy US	290	49	12	8
Venti				
Nonfat Milk	320	58	22	2.5
Whole Milk	440	54	20	20
Soy US	420	72	15	11
Tazo Tea				
Tall	0	0	0	0
Grande	0	0	0	0
Venti	0	0	0	0
Tazo Chai Tea Latte				
Tall				
Nonfat Milk	170	37	6	0
Whole Milk	210	36	6	5
Soy US	190	39	4	2
Grande				
Nonfat Milk	230	51	8	0
Whole Milk	290	50	8	7
Soy US	260	53	6	3
Venti				
Nonfat Milk	300	64	11	0
Whole Milk	360	62	10	9
Soy US	350	72	7	4.5
White Chocolate Mocha (without whipped cream)				
Tall				
Nonfat Milk	260	45	12	4
Whole Milk	320	43	11	12
Soy US	290	47	9	7

	CALORIES	CHO (gm)	PROTEIN (gm)	FAT (gm)
Grande				
Nonfat Milk	340	58	16	5
Whole Milk	410	56	14	15
Soy US	370	62	12	9
Venti				
Nonfat Milk	430	73	20	6
Whole Milk	530	71	18	19
Soy US	470	78	17	13
Cold Beverages				
Iced Caffe Latte				
Tall				
Nonfat Milk	70	11	7	0
Whole Milk	120	10	6	6
Soy US	90	13	5	2.5
Grande				
Nonfat Milk	100	14	9	0
Whole Milk	160	13	8	8
Soy US	120	17	6	3.5
Venti				
Nonfat Milk	130	19	12	0
Whole Milk	210	17	11	10
Soy US	160	23	8	4.5
Iced Caffe Mocha (without whipped cream)				
Tall				
Nonfat Milk	130	27	7	1.5
Whole Milk	170	26	7	6
Soy US	150	28	5	3.5
Grande				
Nonfat Milk	180	36	9	2
Whole Milk	220	35	9	8
Soy US	200	38	7	4.5
Venti				
Nonfat Milk	260	52	13	3.5
Whole Milk	310	51	12	11
Soy US	300	58	10	7
Iced Tazo Chai				
Tall				
Nonfat Milk	170	36	6	0
Whole Milk	200	36	5	5
Soy US	180	38	4	2
Grande				
Nonfat Milk	230	50	8	0
Whole Milk	270	48	7	7
Soy US	250	52	5	3

	CALORIES	CHO (gm)	PROTEIN (gm)	FAT (gm)
Venti				
Nonfat Milk	320	70	11	0
Whole Milk	380	68	10	9
Soy US	350	73	7	4
Frappuccino Blended Coffee				
Coffee				
Tall	190	38	4	2.5
Grande	260	52	5	3.5
Venti	350	69	7	4.5
Mocha (without whipped cream)				
Tall	220	44	5	3
Grande	290	58	6	4
Venti	400	81	8	6
Caramel (without whipped cream)				
Tall	210	43	4	2.5
Grande	280	57	5	3.5
Venti	390	79	7	4.5
Frappuccino Light Blended Coffee				
Coffe				
Tall	110	22	5	1
Grande	150	30	7	1
Venti	200	39	9	1.5
Mocha				
Tall	140	28	5	1.5
Grande	180	36	7	1.5
Venti	250	52	10	2.5
Caramel				
Tall	140	28	5	1.5
Grande	180	36	7	1.5
Venti	250	51	9	2
Extras				
Whipped Cream Topping (No sprinkles or drizzle)				
Cold Beverages				
Tall	90	2	0	9
Grande/Venti	130	2	0	12
Hot Beverages				
All Sizes	100	2	0	9
Flavored Syrup (1 Pump)	20	5	0	0
Flavored Sugar-free Syrup (1 Pump)	0	0	0	0
Mocha Syrup (1 Pump)	25	6	1	0.5

	CALORIES	CHO (gm)	PROTEIN (gm)	FAT (gm)
Subway®				
6" Cold Subs				
Veggie Delite®	230	44	9	3
Turkey breast	280	46	17	4.5
Ham	290	46	18	5
Roast beef	290	45	19	5
Tuna	530	45	22	31
6" Hot Subs				
Roasted chicken breast	330	47	24	5
Steak and cheese	390	48	24	14
Meatball	540	53	23	26
Sweet onion chicken teriyaki	380	59	17	5
Deli Style Sandwiches				
Turkey breast	210	36	12	4
Ham	210	35	11	4
Roast beef	220	35	13	4.5
Tuna	330	36	13	16
Salads				
Veggie Delite®	50	9	2	1
Turkey	100	11	10	2.5
Roasted chicken breast	150	12	16	3
Tuna with cheese	360	12	16	29
Salad Dressings and Sauces				
Fat-free French (1 Pkg.)	70	17	0	0
Fat-free Italian (1 Pkg.)	20	4	0	0
Fat-free Ranch (1 Pkg.)	60	14	0	0
Chipotle Southwest (1.5 T)	90	2	0	9
Fat-free Honey Mustard (1.5 T)	30	7	0	0
Fat-free Sweet Onion (1.5 T)	40	9	0	0
Mayonnaise (1 T)	110	0	0	12
Light mayonnaise (1 T)	50	1	0	5
Taco Bell				
Bean burrito	370	55	14	10
Burrito supreme, beef	390	51	14	18
Burrito supreme, steak	420	50	16	16
Burrito supreme, chicken	410	50	18	14
7 Layer	530	57	18	22
Taco	170	13	8	10
Soft taco, beef	210	21	10	10
Soft taco, chicken	190	19	14	6
Double decker taco	340	39	15	14

FOR   MORE   INFORMATION   .   .   .

Books

Jacobson, M. and Hurley, J. 2002. *Restaurant Confidential.*
    Washington, D.C.: Center for Science in the Public Interest.
Warshaw, H. 2002. *Guide to Healthy Restaurant Eating.* New York:
    McGraw Hill.

Websites

Arby's	http://www.arbys.com
Baja Fresh	http://www.bajafresh.com
Brueggers Bagels	http://www.brueggers.com
Burger King	http://www.burgerking.com
Chick-fil-A	http://www.chick-fil-a.com
Chipotle	http://www.calorieking.com
Cosi	http://www.getcosi.com
Domino's Pizza	http://www.dominos.com
Dunkin Donuts	http://www.dunkindonuts.com
Jamba Juice	http://www.jambajuice.com
Krispy Kreme Doughnuts	http://www.krispykreme.com
McDonald's	http://www.mcdonalds.com
Noodles and company	http://www.calorieking.com
Panera Bread	http://www.panerabread.com
P.F. Chang's	http://www.Pfchangs.com
Quizno's	http://www.calorieking.com
Sbarros	http://www.calorieking.com
Southern Tsunami	http://www.calorieking.com
Subway	http://www.subway.com
Starbucks	http://www.starbucks.com
Taco Bell	http://www.tacobell.com

Nutrition Sense and Nonsense

"Lose five pounds in five days," "amino acid pills will improve your athletic performance," "take vitamin C to prevent colds." Today, there seems to be a dietary solution for whatever ails you. Supplements, weight loss miracles, and "natural" therapies are examples of the increasing number of products or services aimed at helping you be a better you. Do they work? Are they safe?

When it comes to dispensing accurate nutrition advice, there are as many questions about how nutrition affects your health as there are answers, and there are more possibilities for its role in good health than there are proven facts. Some of the claims about nutrition are true. Many, however, are not.

Scientific-sounding studies or "experts" back most of the advice and claims you hear or read about. As you go through this chapter, you'll discover how to determine if they are credible. Your job is to be a skeptic—a free thinker—and to learn how to read between the lines so you can separate factual information from hype, which ultimately means separating helpful information from misinformation that could harm you (see Chart 3–1).

A Taste of Nonsense

Nutrition "solutions" targeted at the college crowd generally focus on improving athletic performance, increasing energy, or losing weight. It may be hard to avoid the sell (it's everywhere), but before you shell out your money and, more important, your health, here's a heads-up on some of the more popular products and claims lurking out there.

Miracle Supplements

Chromium picolinate, creatine, and echinacea are hot right now. The claims made about chromium picolinate are that it increase your energy and helps you to lose weight permanently. Recently, the Federal Trade Commission (a government regulatory agency) stepped in and asked for proof of the stated claims about chromium picolinate. The claims couldn't be substantiated. In other words, it hasn't been shown to help you lose weight or increase your energy. But that hasn't stopped it from becoming a $100 million dollar bestseller.

Creatine is a popular supplement being used by people hoping to increase their muscle mass, strength, and endurance. Only a handful of studies (all of them small) supports this claim. Creatine does appear to help you bulk up. However, it's a transient fix and once you stop using the supplement, it's benefits disappear.

Echinacea is recommended for everything from preventing colds to relieving toothaches. Although it appears to be relatively safe, its efficacy is questionable. But how can one supplement cure so many

---

CHART 3–1

Fact or Fiction?

1. Chocolate and fried foods will give you zits.
3. Eat gelatin for stronger nails.
3. Lose weight quickly.
4. Eating "white" food is bad for you.
5. Athletes need more protein than non-athletes.
6. A regular fasting day will help "detox" your body.
7. Sugar makes you hyperactive.
8. Regular exercise gives you a "high."
9. Eating chicken soup when you are sick makes you feel better.
10. Vitamins and minerals—more are better.

Answers

1. **Fiction.** Although eating a high-fat diet may be bad for your health, your diet has little to do with acne. Hormonal changes, stress, and certain environmental changes are more likely to influence the process that causes pimples to develop.
2. **Fiction.** Based on a theory that gelatin is a good protein that will improve blood flow to the nails, the science to support this just isn't there.
3. **Fiction.** Nothing more needs to be said. Permanent weight loss is neither quick nor easy. So anything promising to deliver dramatic results fast is pulling a fast one on you.
4. **Fiction.** Yes, whole grain or "brown" breads, cereals, pasta, and rice do contain more nutrients and fiber. They are healthier, but the white stuff won't kill you. It just doesn't pack the same nutrients bite for bite.
5. **Fact.** A slightly larger amount of protein is needed to build muscle. However, you can get this easily by eating a well-balanced diet, and protein supplements generally aren't necessary.
6. **Fiction.** Although an occasional fast isn't harmful, our bodies are very efficient machines and have the ability to clear substances out naturally, without fasting.
7. **Fiction.** Eating a diet high in sugar is not nourishing because it doesn't provide a balance of nutrients. While sugar does supply immediate fuel to your body, no studies support the notion that this actually "revs" you up.
8. **Fact.** Exercising regularly for a certain period of time can give you a sense of well- being because of the release of endorphins. Even if you don't feel "high," exercise should make your body feel good.
9. **Fact.** This has actually been tested and proven. Although no one can figure out why, a little chicken soup is good medicine.
10. **Fiction.** This type of thinking can get you into big trouble. Your body needs only minute amounts of vitamins and minerals. By getting them through food, you're unlikely to get too much. However, in pill form, you can overdose on some, even if they're natural. The best way to get what you need is from food first.

things? Like so many things in life, if it seems too good to be true, it probably is.

THE BOTTOM LINE: When a label or advertisement says it can cure many things or that it can significantly change your life, beware. Miracle discoveries and revolutionary findings rarely occur. It takes more than pills or potions to make an impact on health issues such as fatigue and obesity. Vitamins, minerals, herbs, and other supplements like chromium picolinate, creatine, and echinicea should be used carefully, cautiously, and ideally with your doctor's blessing.

Dieting Gimmicks

It's gimmicks galore in the dieting industry. Eat grapefruit to burn more calories, avoid bread to stay thin, flush fat from your body when you eat fruit with meat are just a few of the millions of tricks people are pushing to "help" you lose weight. The weight loss industry is beyond gigantic; Americans spend at least $33 billion dollars a year on products and services that promise a slimmer and trimmer way of life.

THE BOTTOM LINE: You can cut through the clutter of claims if you remember:

- All food contains calories.

  If you eat more than your body burns, you'll gain weight. It doesn't matter if those calories are from peanut butter or from cucumbers.

- Nothing you eat burns calories.

  Eating grapefruit before a meal is good advice because it's a nutritious fruit, it contains only a small number of calories, and it's filling. But its ability to burn any other calories you eat is wishful thinking.

- No magic potion, pill, or machine can help you lose weight quickly and effortlessly.

  "Diet drugs" have been around for a while. To date, their long-term success is questionable, and it's too early to tell what the long-term side effects will be. Short-term complications such as heart valve problems, have already surfaced. These products should only be used if they are prescribed and monitored by a medical doctor who is familiar with you and your family's medical history.

- Foods can be eaten in just about any combination.

They do not need to be strategically paired. Every few years, a new "food-combining" diet appears on the scene claiming that you should or shouldn't eat certain types of foods at the same time. Food combining, as sexy as it sounds, lacks scientific evidence.

Cellulite Fixes

Cellulite is a non-medical term used to describe the "cottage cheese"-like appearance of skin on certain parts of the body, most often in the thighs and butt. Cellulite is nothing more than plain old fat accumulated under the skin. Unfortunately, skin texture and genetics make some individuals more susceptible to the unsightly waffled look than others.

THE BOTTOM LINE: The best way to minimize cellulite is to exercise regularly. Wraps, machines, and supplements won't remove a thing.

Natural and Organic

If it's "natural," it must be healthy! Right? Sounds reasonable, but the term "natural" is not firmly defined by the federal agencies that regulate the use of other terms, such as "low-fat," "fresh," or "light." "Natural" is open to interpretation and is used and abused by manufacturers and advertisers.

THE BOTTOM LINE: Natural is not necessarily healthier, lower in calories, or tastier. Read the fine print on labels—don't be sold on natural alone (see Chart 3–2).

The term "organic" simply describes how a food—whether it's produce, meat, grains, or dairy foods—is produced. The Organic

CHART 3–2

Natural Snack Food vs. Traditional Snack Food

	FOOD LABEL FOR NATURAL VEGGIE STIX	FOOD LABEL FOR POTATO CHIPS
Serving Size	1 oz.	1 oz.
Calories	140	150
Total grams of fat (gm)	6	8.5
Total Carbohydrate (gm)	19	16
Protein (gm)	1	2

Foods Production Act of 1998 requires that any food sold or labeled as "organically grown" or "organically produced" must meet specific growing, producing, or processing standards. Organic foods won't necessarily contain less fat, taste better, or be more nutritious.

Organic farming is "environmentally friendly." Because organic foods lack the chemical residues found in some pesticides, they may offer long-term health benefits to your body.

Now It's Your Turn—Figure Out Science on Your Own

You can wade through the health information in magazines, newspapers, and the Internet, and you can decipher fact from fiction. Just ask yourself a few simple questions. The following guidelines will help you evaluate what you read, what you see, and what you hear.

Look closely at who is saying it.

Credentials are tricky. In some states, anyone can call him or herself a "nutritionist," in other states the term is regulated. Some states have licensing boards. The initials L.D. (Licensed Dietitian) or L.N. (Licensed Nutritionist) after one's name mean that the person has met criteria established by the state for licensing dietitians and nutritionists. A Registered Dietitian (R.D.) has met criteria established by the American Dietetic Association, the largest and most recognized credentialing organization for nutrition professionals. To muddy the waters even more, one can buy bogus nutrition credentials bought from "diploma mills"—organizations that award degrees without requiring students to meet standards accepted by accredited two- and four-year colleges and universities. These organizations are contributing to the proliferation of so-called "experts."

Evaluate all the information, not just the headlines.

If the information is based on the results of one study, beware. Look at how many people participated in the study. A study conducted on a small sample of people must be capable of being reproduced with a different group. Was the study done on people similar to you? Better still, was the study done on humans? Although animal studies are valid, they don't necessarily give you conclusive information that can be applied to humans. Do the claims rely solely on testimonials from "happy" customers? That's not an objective criterion, and it presents too many questions.

Read between the lines.

Studies can be reported in such a way that findings sound reasonable, but on further investigation, are actually misleading. For instance, a study that states a particular vitamin "may" prevent cancer is not saying it "does" cure cancer. Other wordsmithing to watch for—when reports "suggest" a cure, they're not saying there is a cure. The term "contributes to" such as grilling meat contributes to cancer, does not necessarily mean it "causes" the disease.

Avoid cure-all products.

One product or therapy promising to "cure" many different ailments should always be suspect. Non-specific complaints such as fatigue and problems such as obesity and depression require multi-faceted approaches to treatment. But, because these problems are so all-encompassing, they are easy targets for a scam. It's unlikely that one simple solution will ever "fix" any of these problems.

Know the buzzwords.

"Complementary," "integrative," and "alternative" medicine is gaining significant support. While there's a lot to be learned about a more holistic approach to health and disease, keep in mind that all that is "natural" is not necessarily safe. Herbs, vitamins, and other "natural" supplements are not risk-free. In fact, since many natural supplements lack product standards, their quality and content vary tremendously. When supplements and vitamins are used in large doses, they also act more like drugs than vitamins. Self-prescribing large doses of vitamins and other supplements can be just as dangerous and life threatening as self-medicating with prescription drugs.

Pay attention to who is footing the bill for research.

If a study is supported by a certain industry or product, watch for biases in the conclusions and recommendations. Likewise, if you go to a health professional who is making a profit by selling vitamins, supplements, or other products, look carefully and skeptically at any advice given about using these products.

Cyber-Health

The Internet has become a big player in "promoting" nutrition information and products. With powerful search engines, you can simply type in a keyword such as "diet," and be inundated with more information than you could ever want. Use the same evaluation guidelines listed above.

Check the information for its source and advice. If you're encouraged to buy a product, find out how the site is funded. If it just happens to be funded by a company that has a relationship with the product, investigate further.

If the site is an institution or is nationally recognized such as the American Dietetic Association—you're in luck. If it's the National Center for Dieting—you are not; it's fictitious. How do you know? Check beyond the site.

An on-line rating and review guide, www.navigator.tufts.edu, was developed by Tufts University School of Nutrition Science and Policy. It provides an unbiased, educated rating and review system that combs through the daunting number of nutrition-based sites. Tufts' nutrition-ists rate sites from corporate, academic, and government sources based on content usability, depth, and accuracy of nutrition information as criteria.

THE BOTTOM LINE: There are no quick fixes to better health. Unsubstantiated claims from unqualified individuals are hard to resist, especially if you're struggling with a chronic problem. But before you give your body and wallet to the next "great idea," investigate for more details. And remember . . . if it sounds too good to be true, it probably is!

PART II
Weighing In

The "Freshman 15"

High on the anxiety meter for first-year college students is the fear of "the freshman 15"—the notorious weight gain that often occurs within the first several months of arriving on campus. Putting on pounds is a pretty common problem for the soon-to-be well-educated. The good news is that it doesn't have to be a problem for you.

Like a kid in a candy store, your first encounter with mass quantities of ready-to-eat dorm food and the availability of food 24 hours a day may seem pretty enticing. There are unlimited choices of food and no parents to tell you what, how much, or when to eat. Indulge too often, and the result can be extra weight to lug around campus. You can tighten your belt, however, if you're aware of the situations that can cause you to gain weight, and if you're willing to take some simple steps toward managing them.

Obstacles to Eating Well

It's a jungle out there. You're new to campus life, you probably don't know many people, and you're far away from home. Everything is foreign, well almost everything. Food is a familiar companion, a wonderful coping device in the midst of chaos.

Below are some of the common pitfalls that cause you to gain weight and some useful strategies for avoiding them.

Whacked-out Schedules

Face it . . . college life is different than the regime you left at home, where you probably ate at regular mealtimes, slept at regular hours, and followed a fairly regular routine. Now class schedules change often, all-nighters are all too frequent, and scheduled breakfast, lunch, and dinner are a thing of the past. This departure from the norm can destroy your diet. To avoid problems, try the following:

- Respect the importance of mealtimes, and put yourself on a schedule.

  Meals are your fuel, and your body likes to be fed every three to five hours. Your body performs its best when it is "fed" early and regularly. Eating regularly—every three to five hours—makes it easier to avoid the out-of-control eating that occurs when you get really hungry.

- Give up grazing and eat meals instead.

  "Grazing," the act of eating small portions of food continuously rather than full meals, isn't a substitute for a well-rounded meal. Eating meals is different from grazing. If you don't make it a point to sit down and eat, you'll find yourself eating a handful of pretzels here, some fries there. Even if what you grab is "good" food, grazing is not going to satisfy your hunger, and you're much more likely to overeat.

- Eat shortly after you wake up.

  Many opt for sleeping, rather than breakfast, proud they saved calories by eliminating a meal. The reality is that without breakfast,
  those "saved" calories are more than made up for later in the day.
  Breakfast doesn't have to be at 7 A.M., but eating within an hour of
  waking is important. It revs up your metabolism, slips your brain
  into gear, and helps control "pigging out" later in the day.

- Choose decent late-night snacks.

  Contrary to all you've heard, eating late at night is no more likely
  to add pounds to your body than eating during the day. If you're
  a night owl or you're going to be up into the wee hours of the
  morning, plan to eat a snack. Remember the three- to five-hour
  rule. If you eat dinner at 6:30 P.M. and remain awake until 2 A.M.,
  another meal is in order. Meal patterns for various schedules are
  suggested in Chart 4–1 and can help you discover a new routine
  to work with your new lifestyle.

So Many Choices

Eating in the cafeteria is like eating in a restaurant. It offers foods
you may never have had at home and in quantities you might never
have seen before. Instead of Mom or Dad leading the way, it's up to
you what you'll eat, when you'll eat, and how much you'll eat. If you
know how to eat in a healthy way, you'll know which foods can help
keep your waist in check and which ones may lead to weight gain (see
Chapter 1). If you don't know which foods are a part of a healthy diet,
you increase your chances of packing on the pounds. To avoid problems, try to:

- Make two trips through the line instead of one.

  Go back for dessert after you finish the meal—you'll be full by
  then, so what looks like a good dessert or how much dessert you
  want to eat may be different than when you went through the line
  hungry.

CHART 4–1

Flexible Eating Schedules

Here are meal patterns for every schedule. No matter what your schedule is, you can create a pattern to keep you on track.

EARLY CLASS DAY

7:00 – 9:00 A.M.	Breakfast:	2 cereal bars and skim milk
11:30 – 1:00 P.M.	Lunch:	Turkey sandwich, small bag of chips, fruit
5:00 – 6:00 P.M.	Dinner:	Salad veggies, baked potato, baked chicken, fruit
9:30 –11:00 P.M.	Snack:	2 slices plain pizza

Total: 1936 calories. 107 gm protein, 73 gm fat, 223 gm carbohydrate

5 DAY

8:00 – 9:30 A.M.	Breakfast:	Special K, milk, banana, toast with spread
12:00 – 1:30 P.M.	Lunch:	Veggie burger on a bun, tomato soup, apple
4:00 – 5:00 P.M.	Snack:	Fruit smoothie
7:00 – 8:00 P.M.	Dinner:	Pasta with sauce, roll, salad, skim milk, brownie

Total: 1849 calories. 68 gm protein, 49 gm fat, 276 gm carbohydrate

WEEKEND

1:00 – 2:30 P.M.	Brunch:	Scrambled eggs, juice, English muffin with spread
3:00 – 4:30 P.M.	Snack:	Skim milk latte and muffin
5:30 – 7:30 P.M.	Dinner:	Grilled chicken sandwich, salad, dressing
10:30 –12:00 A.M.	Snack:	2 slices pizza

Total: 1633 calories. 89 gm protein, 62 gm fat, 188 gm carbohydrate

SLEEPING IN

12:30 – 2:00 P.M.	Lunch:	Veggie and cheese wrap
4:00 – 5:00 P.M.	Snack:	Bowl of soup
6:00 – 8:00 P.M.	Dinner:	Stir-fried chicken with rice and vegetables, fruit salad, cookie
12:00 – 2:00 A.M.	Snack:	Bagel with light cream cheese, juice

Total: 1593 calories. 83 gm protein, 31 gm fat, 246 gm carbohydrate

ON THE FLY

10:00 –11:00 A.M.		Bagel with light cream cheese, coffee
2:00 – 3:00 P.M.		Bean burrito
7:30 – 8:30 P.M.		Pizza, side salad
12:00 – 1:00 A.M.		Cereal and milk

Total: 1690 calories. 75 gm protein, 46 gm fat, 247 gm carbohydrate

(Beverages as indicated or water)

- Commit to at least one serving of fruit and one serving of vegetables at both lunch and dinner.

  Unadorned, they are low in calories and fat and fairly filling.

- Balance your choices.

  Remember the pyramid and plan your meals. If your options are pasta, potatoes, and bread choose one serving, not all three. Look for some fruit, veggies, and/or salad. **Add some protein**. Obvious choices are lean meat, fish, or poultry. However, if what's available looks unappetizing, hard-boiled eggs, cottage cheese, canned tuna, or beans will meet your needs. You can always add a glass of skim milk, too, for high-quality protein. Use high-fat condiments sparingly. A spoonful of salad dressing adds taste, a ladle adds unwanted calories. If you choose dessert at lunch, skip it at dinner. You can eat well, even in the dining hall. It's a matter of knowing healthy vs. unhealthy and looking beyond the junk to the good stuff. It really is there.

So Little Control

The foods you eat at home are usually prepared the way you like them. Chances are your cafeteria is not privy to that information. Some of the foods offered may be loaded with fat or served with high-calorie sauces. Portions may be significantly larger than what was served at home. Some foods might taste so good that you just can't get enough of them. Others taste so bland that you overeat until you feel stuffed, still searching for something that hits the spot. Some suggested solutions are:

- Go for plain food.

  If you're not sure what ingredients are used in "mystery" dishes such as a casserole or stew, opt for the more basically prepared dishes like baked or broiled chicken or even a burger (see Chapter 2 for entrées that pass the test.)

- Cruise through the cafeteria before making any selections.

  Choose the healthiest offerings available. Check with the staff serving the food; they may be willing to accommodate a few special requests. Some reasonable ones are:

Can you serve sauces/dressing on the side?

Do you have plain, steamed veggies available?

Will you serve baked potatoes or sweet potatoes in addition to other potatoes?

Do you have vinegar, olive oil, lemon, mustard, salsa and low cal salad dressings available?

Is ice water available?

Do you have skim, soy or lactaid milk?

Can you have hard-boiled eggs, cottage cheese, tofu, and water-packed tuna at the salad bar?

Will you serve smaller portions?

Will you offer yogurt at all meals?

Do you have veggie burgers?

Can you offer plain grilled chicken breasts?

Emotional and Non-Hunger Eating

College life (especially freshman year) is a roller coaster of emotions—boredom, stress, loneliness, among others. Food can serve as a great distracter, comfort or social crutch. Food serves many other functions in addition to satisfying hunger. Using food to cope, celebrate, relax, or procrastinate are all examples of non-hunger eating. All of us occasionally eat when we're not hungry, but the ability to manage non-hunger eating is key to avoiding weight gain.

Before you eat, decide whether you truly are hungry. Are you eating food because your body needs food, or for some other reason? Eating when you're not hungry will happen, so be prepared.

- Become aware of the non-hunger cues that motivate you to eat.

  When the cues hit, give yourself an arbitrary time—say five minutes—to determine if you really want to eat. If you still want to eat, set a realistic portion of food, such as a coffee mug of pretzels in front of you instead of an entire box of crackers, cookies, or chips. Sit down, focus only on eating rather than eating and watching TV, or eating and talking on the phone. Inattentive eating translates into hundreds of unaccounted calories.

- Have low-calorie munchies on hand.

The food on Chart 4–2 will never satisfy you if you're hungry, but they can help you manage non-hunger eating. Because all foods have calories, regularly indulging in even lower-calorie choices will still add up.

CHART 4–2

Lower-Calorie Non-Hunger Munchies to Have on Hand

Baby carrots	Tootsie Roll Pops
Popcorn	Sugar Daddy
Fresh and canned fruit	Herbal tea
Fresh, frozen, or canned vegetables	Hot cocoa
Frozen fruit pops	

- Don't resort to "fat-free" or "low carb" when you're trying to cope with non-hunger eating.

Fat-free or low carb is not calorie-free, and you're more likely to give yourself permission to overindulge (see Chart 4–3).

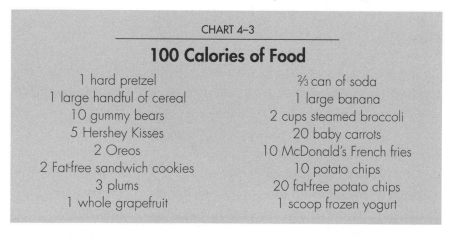

CHART 4–3

100 Calories of Food

1 hard pretzel	⅔ can of soda
1 large handful of cereal	1 large banana
10 gummy bears	2 cups steamed broccoli
5 Hershey Kisses	20 baby carrots
2 Oreos	10 McDonald's French fries
2 Fat-free sandwich cookies	10 potato chips
3 plums	20 fat-free potato chips
1 whole grapefruit	1 scoop frozen yogurt

- To manage the food/mood connection, create a list of at least three things you can do instead of eating when you're bored, stressed, tired, or sad.

Create your list now (see Chart 4–4) so that you're armed and ready when the moods strike. Some possibilities for the list are

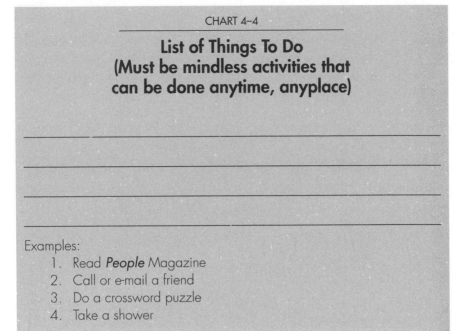

CHART 4–4

**List of Things To Do
(Must be mindless activities that
can be done anytime, anyplace)**

Examples:
1. Read *People* Magazine
2. Call or e-mail a friend
3. Do a crossword puzzle
4. Take a shower

reading a favorite magazine, calling a friend, taking a shower, or doing a crossword puzzle.

Recreational Eating

The social aspect of eating is enormously important. Dining halls, food courts, and campus eateries are not only places to eat, but places to hang out. Sitting around and eating is a popular activity in college.

Sometimes just being with certain people can be a cue to eat. For example, do you have "eating buddies" i.e., friends you can always depend on to order a gooey dessert or loaded nachos? Simply being aware of the relationship can put you in charge of the situation.

It may be tough to sit around a table and talk without food in front of you. With frozen yogurt or ice cream just steps away from where you're sitting, and your friends lingering around the table munching on stuff, that extra scoop is hard to resist.

- Take deliberate steps to end your meal.

  Brush your teeth, suck on a mint, chew gum, or drink a glass of water to cue yourself that the meal is over.

- When you're done eating, get up and remove your plate.

Any food left on your plate will surely be consumed if it sits in front of you long enough.

- Create alternative activities.

Next time the "munch bunch" gets together, bring something else to do while they're eating or suggest that the group do something else, such as taking a walk, sitting outside, etc.

The Drinking Man's (or Woman's) Diet

Drinking is alive and well on college campuses (see Chapter 11 for more information on drinking). Large quantities of alcohol equate to large numbers of calories, which often leads to rapid weight gain. In addition to drinking your calories, the "munchies" often take over with a vengeance, and lots of less than healthy food sneak their way into your body (see Chart 4–5).

- Pay attention to the calories in alcohol.

Drinking calories add up very quickly.

- Never drink on an empty stomach.

Although you may want to "save" your calories for those in beer, this could be particularly dangerous. Drinking on an empty stomach will lead to faster absorption of the alcohol and could present serious problems.

- Alternate each beverage with water or seltzer.

Filling in with these fluids allows you to have something in your hand and space out your alcohol intake.

- Dilute mixers with water or seltzer.

It isn't only the calories in the alcohol; blenderized drinks and drinks mixed with juice and soda add even more calories.

- It is always acceptable to decline a drink.

CHART 4–5

How Many Calories Are You Drinking?

BEVERAGE	CALORIES
12 oz. beer	140–150
6 pack beer	840–900
12 oz. lite beer	95–105
12 oz. ultra beer	95
4 oz. red wine	90–120
4 oz. white wine	80–120
1.5 oz. shot of liquor	100
7 oz. mixed drink	175
12 oz. blender drink	725

And munching?

3 handfuls of mixed nuts	525
1 order of nachos, split with three others	300
½ bag of baked Lays	420
3 potato skins	400
Personal pizza	500–600
⅓ box of hard pretzels	500–600
1 pint of frozen yogurt	400–600
1 bag of M&M's	230
2 large chocolate chip cookies	500

Bottom Line . . . Faking Out the Freshman 15

With the amount of time you will probably spend around food, the lack of a routine schedule, and the new opportunities to eat and drink as much as you like, the freshman 15 is a real possibility. The three most common reasons for the weight gain are:

- Lack of a consistent schedule;
- Excessive alcohol intake;
- 24-hour-a-day eating.

If you prepare yourself to manage the array of food choices available, set an eating schedule for yourself, decrease high calorie partying, and develop strategies for dealing with non-hunger eating, you can avoid the weight gain.

CHAPTER

5

Reality Dieting

The "freshman 15," as discussed in Chapter 4, is frequently caused by a handful of factors.

- An unlimited amount of food available nearly every hour of the day
- A certain amount of comfort in eating familiar foods when everything and everyone is new
- An overindulgence of alcohol
- A more sedentary way of life (at least for some students)

So, what do you do if the pounds start piling on?

If you are like 45 million other Americans, you go on a diet. Eager to believe that the latest diet popularized by a celebrity, a doctor or your best friend is the answer, you get caught up in the hype. There are plenty of options to choose from. More than half of the 50 best-selling diet books *ever written* have been published since 1999.

Why are Americans packing on the pounds if so many best-selling diets exist? The answer: Diets don't work. They offer hope, but they deliver primarily empty promises. And to add insult to injury, the more we diet, the fatter we are likely to get.

Recycled Diets

Americans buy diet books, products and gimmicks to the tune of **$46 billion** a year. Looking at the success rate of most of these products, it's probably not money well spent.

Besides being ineffective, many diet concepts are cyclical. Wait long enough, and you see recurring plans and notions pitched. They simply sport a new face or offer a different twist to grab your attention. (Chart 5–1) For example, high-protein, low carbohydrate plans have been in vogue over the past few years. They were all the rage in the 1970s too. They didn't have staying power then and they lack it now as well.

Certain foods or groups of foods fall in and out of favor too. Currently the focus is on low carbohydrate foods, yet just a few short years ago, carbohydrates could do no wrong—fat was the "forbidden fruit." Today the tables are turned. Fat, or at least certain types of fat, have gained more favor and some kinds of carbohydrates are being shunned. And, to further muddy the waters, somewhere in between nutrition gospel and trendy plans are the perennial programs such as Weight Watchers, Jenny Craig and Slim Fast.

Typical "Diets"

Diets are packaged in many different and sometimes innovative ways, yet they are still *diets*. Most tend to have a hook—something

CHART 5-1

Decades of Dieting

TIMELINE	THE SKINNY ON THE DIET	A REALITY CHECK
1960s		
Weight Watchers	Weight Watchers was started by founder Jean Nidetch, who began inviting women into her home to discuss the best way to lose weight. Today, the program has millions of followers who buy books, food products, join, rejoin and can now do it all online.	From a nutritional standpoint, the diet is balanced. It teaches people portion control, is adaptable for different populations including vegetarians and pregnant women. Problem: it still uses a "diet" mentality meaning people are either on it or off it. If you can take what you learn from Weight Watchers and make it more flexible, the plan is acceptable for the long run.
The Stillman Diet	**Dr. Stillman's** *The Doctor's Quick Weight Loss Diet* was a first of the low carb, high protein diets to go mainstream. He pushed protein, believing that it requires more calories to digest it.	Very restrictive. This high protein diet had many side effects including weakness, bad breath, nausea and constipation. Once you got rid of carbs, you got rid of a lot of calories. No longer a popular diet—it's been replaced several times over by other high protein, low carb diets.
Twiggy	The first model embodying waif-like thinness hits the pages of Seventeen Magazine.	Young women continue to emulate unrealistic body images. Once an anomaly, today nearly all models mirror her image fueling the body dissatisfaction prevalent among young women.
1970s		
U.S. Dietary Goals	The first federal document released to the public that looked at the relationship between what we eat and how it affects the risk for various diseases such as heart disease, diabetes and certain types of cancers.	Replaced by the Dietary Guidelines which are now updated about every five years. If followed, they can be the right way to eat to stay healthy and fit. Unfortunately, they lack the sizzle and mystique that capture public interest and attract followers.

TIMELINE	THE SKINNY ON THE DIET	A REALITY CHECK
Diet Centers and Nutrisystem	Commercial diet programs patterned after Weight Watchers but with more rigid calorie plans. Originally storefront settings, you can now access both online. (Diet Centers still has on site counseling.) Both recommend their own products and Diet Centers sells "thermogenic" diet supplements. They are expensive and leave little room for normalizing food intake when you "stop".	No one can follow these severely restrictive meal plans for any length of time. Another example of "on a diet you lose, off the diet you gain it back". Plus, they tend to be expensive.
Atkins Diet	**Dr. Robert Atkins** introduces his low-carb **Diet Revolution,** encouraging dieters to drastically cut carbs and eat more protein and fat. Claims the body will burn stored fat for calories and weight loss will result. Also claims you will never feel hungry on this plan.	See info under revised plan, 2000.
Scarsdale Diet	**Dr. Tarnower** introduces **The Complete Scarsdale Medical Diet.** Another version of high protein, low carb concept, with very specific meal plans mapped out.	Followers lost weight for the 14 days they stayed on this very low calorie diet, but regained it when done. With the death of Dr. Tarnower, this diet fell by the wayside and is no longer a player in the crowded diet industry.
Pritikin Diet	**Dr. Pritikin** introduces the **Pritikin Program for Diet and Exercise.** Philosophy originally developed at the Pritikin Longevity Centers where people checked in to become healthier, Nathan Pritikin then went on to write books to carry the message to the public. The diet mantra prescribes eliminating foods which are "dense" in calories and eating a diet rich in fruits and vegetables. Diet is extremely low in fat and vegetables. Diet is extremely low in fat and lead the way to the low fat, high fiber, high carb diets.	See info under revised plan, 1990s.

TIMELINE	THE SKINNY ON THE DIET	A REALITY CHECK
1980s		
Liquid diets	**The Cambridge Diet** and **Optifast** diet encourage millions to exist on low-calorie liquid protein drinks. They were in popularity after fatal heart attacks are reported and high profile personalities who once touted the benefits of the diet promptly regain all lost weight.	One could never exist on these diets. Too limiting, too monotonous, no direction for how to reintroduce food. No discussion on lifestyle/behavioral change. Nasty side effects including bad breath. Offered short term solution, with dismal long term success.
Celebrity Diets	Celebrities advertise their way to maintain/lose weight. **The Beverly Hills Diet** by actress **Judy Mazel** is introduced. The diet, based on eating only fruit is quickly abandoned after reports of serious side effects. Other celebrities such as Oprah's trainer and chef and Suzanne Somers quickly add their names to the list of "do it my way" and publish bestselling diet books for years to come. **Richard Simmons** and **Jane Fonda** produce exercise videos.	The Beverly Hills Diet by Judy Mazel was based on nutrition myths. It did pave the way for celebrities to take advantage of the hot diet marketplace. Most of these plans are based on anecdotal stories of success with little or no science to support the claims made.
Meal replacements: Jenny Craig/ Slim Fast	Meal replacements take the guesswork out of what and how much to eat. Purchasing food packages and being able to "check in" with support networks are appealing.	Ditto to the assessment of diet centers in the 70s.
Fat Phobia	Fat becomes the target of our weight and health concerns. Fat-free products flood the marketplace. Food companies emphasize low-fat virtues, but in many cases calories in product remain the same.	The U.S. government suggested Americans lower their fat intake to minimize weight gain and reduce the risk for heart disease. The food industry followed suit. Consumers saw "fat-free" as permission to eat, actually overeat. Even though a food was fat-free, the calories content remained the same or in some instances was higher. Many people actually gained weight from fat-free foods.

TIMELINE	THE SKINNY ON THE DIET	A REALITY CHECK
1990s		
Pritikin Diet	**Robert Pritikin**, son of Dr. Nathan Pritikin, publishes a new version of his father's low-fat weight loss diet, **Pritikin Centers** open up around the country allowing people to check in (at a hefty price) to "get healthy". Diet is tweaked but is basically a very low fat, high carb diet focusing on the importance of choosing foods which are not calorie dense. Think apples over cookies.	According to the Pritikin plan taking the fat out of the diet is key to weight loss and heart health. Too hard to follow because it does not allow for eating away from home in any practical way. A commitment to a dramatic change in life style is needed to make this diet work.
Eat More, Weigh Less	**Dr. Dean Ornish** publishes his version of a low-fat diet, taking it one step further than Pritikin: a vegetarian diet. Receives high marks for effectiveness but few fans can hang on because diet is quite rigid and following it for the long term is a challenge.	Follows the same theory that slashing fat is key to weight loss. This diet is a more rigid version of Pritikin and unnecessarily restricts healthy sources of animal protein including poultry and fish.
The Zone	A new take on the high protein diet. Plan is complex: 40/30/30 ration emphasizing 40% carbs, 30% protein, 30% fat. Emphasizes lean protein and low sugar foods.	Cut through all of the complicated information and guidelines and the bottom line for this diet is fewer calories. The total calorie intake is about 1,500, a number at which most people will likely lose weight. Although it primarily relies on healthy foods, it makes eating way too complicated. Not scientifically valid.
Sugar Busters	According to this diet sugar is toxic. Eating sugar causes the body to increase the release of insulin which prevents people from losing weight. Recommends all sugars be eliminated from the diet. Recommends eating a higher level of fat than most other diets. Limits carbs and protein to 30% of calories	Eat a lot of sugars, then remove them from your diet, chances are you will lose weight. Though the diet suggests differently, sugar is not toxic, it simply tastes good so we tend to eat more than we should! When evaluated, total calories suggested came to less than 1,000/day, which is way too low for anyone to follow for any length of time.

TIMELINE	THE SKINNY ON THE DIET	A REALITY CHECK
Protein Power	**Michael Eades** follows the high protein trend, suggesting that our bodies have no need for carbs. Calls for severely restricting carbs with remainder of calories coming from protein and fat.	When one food group is severely restricted, chances are you are going to lose weight. No magic, just fewer calories. The problem is, most people won't want to go through life without including their favorite foods.
The New Beverly Hills Diet	**Judy Mazel** tries again.	Not much new about it. Same hype, little science.
Fen-Phen	Diet pill combo becomes widely used and abused. Helps many people lose weight but recalled after takers experience heart problems.	While this particular combo was over-prescribed, there are some situations where medications might be indicated for weight loss. However, taking drugs for anything requires expert evaluation and monitoring by a qualified health care provider.
2000s		
Carbohydrate "addicts"	Carbohydrate modifications and importance of paying attention to the **glycemic index** (how quickly certain foods raise the level of sugar circulating in the blood) in foods is popularized. Claims overweight people are addicted to carbs.	While there might be something of value in knowing the glycemic index of foods, and some people may find it easier to lose weight if they avoid those foods with high glycemic index, the idea of carbohydrate addiction is a popular myth. You lose weight on this diet because you eat less calorically dense foods.
Atkins Diet	**Dr. Atkins** reintroduces his **New Diet Revolution**. As a country we grow fatter and more desperate. Coming off of the fat free decade, we are ready for something new.	The induction phase of the diet is only about 1,000 calories. Regardless of where those 1,000 calories come from (carbs or protein) chances are good you will always lose weight. It's the calorie level not the source of calories that yield the weight loss. It is very restrictive, making it easy to follow in the beginning. The restrictive nature becomes monotonous. Once you stray and eat the maligned carbs, weight loss stops.

TIMELINE	THE SKINNY ON THE DIET	A REALITY CHECK
South Beach Diet	**Dr. Agatston,** a Florida cardiologist, introduces a low-fat, low-carb, high protein diet. Seen as an improvement over Atkins because it allows dieters to eat some carbs.	Like Atkins, South Beach cuts out most carbs, therefore cutting out many calories. Initially, the calorie level of this diet is in the 1,200 range. Chances are you'd lose weight regardless of where those 1200 calories came from. Because it does emphasize "better fat" and in second and final phase, some carbs are introduced, it is viewed as healthier version of the standard high protein diets. But it's still a diet whose success is based on the elimination of a whole food group.
Eat Right 4 Your Type	A new gimmick in the dieting world suggesting that your blood type determines the type of diet you should follow. Diets vary depending on blood type, but all plans emphasize a particular food group, thus limiting calories.	Calories are slashed. This time it depends on your blood type. No science supports the premise that blood type has a role in weight.
Fat Flush Plan	The hook is the need to detoxify the liver and lymph system. The plan (book) then morphs into a high protein diet with an emphasis on decreasing "insulin raising carbs".	A diet which draws on old diet folklore, the bottom line being less calories.
Dr. Phil's Ultimate Weight Solution.	Diet is about eating lean protein; limits high calorie sweets. It is sprinkled with Dr. Phil's lifestyle changes including importance of self-control, taking charge of impulse eating and importance of exercise.	The diet relies on mostly healthy foods. His twist is his coaching you through a low-cal diet, lifestyle changes that are necessary for permanent weight loss success and a "can do" attitude. His "get real" attitude is real: losing weight and keeping it off is difficult but possible.

to intrigue or capture your interest such as restricting a certain food or mandating various "rules" of how and when to eat. Most diets will cause you to lose weight because you are eating fewer calories than what you are used to consuming. In fact, look at the nutritional analysis of popular diets found in chart 5–2. Most plans are very similar in calories. However, almost without exception these diets lack the ability to help you sustain the weight you lose. They are effective on the front end because you become focused on following specific directions and are motivated to get results, yet their restrictive nature or monotony make long-term compliance a challenge.

People like typical diets because they offer "**a plan.**" The plan tells you what to eat, how much to eat and when to eat, leaving little room to think or stray. But, temptations exist and trouble ensues when (not if) you find you wish to eat something that's not part of the plan.

CHART 5-2

What's in the Diet?

DIET	AVERAGE CALORIE INTAKE	% FAT	% CHO	% PROTEIN
Atkins	1400–1500	60%	10%	30%
Zone	1400–1600	30%	40%	30%
South Beach (phase 1)	1400–1500	50%	15%	35%
Weight Watchers	1400–1500	25%	55%	20%
Jenny Craig	1400–1500	20%	60%	20%
Ornish	1400-1500	<10%	75%	15–20%

*average amounts based on analyzing several days of each plan

Why Diets Don't Work

Diets fail for many reasons.

- They provide external controls, dictating what, how much and when you can eat yet ignore internal controls such as hunger, fullness and satiety. They do not address issues of emotional eating or valid reasons for non-hunger eating—two very influential factors in what and how people eat.

- They give lip service to lifestyle changes, but those changes are impractical or provide inadequate instruction that will allow you to implement the real changes necessary for permanent weight loss.
- They are not individualized. It has become abundantly clear that the one-size-fits-all approach to health and dieting does not work. Individual interests, needs and events in life make it impossible to use the cookie-cutter approach to dieting and expect it to succeed.
- They overlook the boredom factor. It happens yet few plans offer tools to cope with monotony. When you "go off" the diet, for a meal, a night or a week, you feel like you've blown it. Picking up the pieces seems overwhelming and can trigger the beginning of the end.
- They are too low in calories, making it difficult to stick with the plan for any length of time. No matter how you dress up a diet, it is designed to have you eat less, which of course, is necessary to lose weight. But restrictive eating will only work for so long. You will crave, binge and overeat. That is the natural consequence of eating too little and the set up for a lifelong battle with food.

Perhaps there is something to be learned from each diet. But for this learning experience, it's better to save your money and stay on the sidelines. Regardless of the nutritional adequacy of any diet, the dieting mentality of going on and off a diet is never going to be your answer to permanent weight loss. It's just going to be a temporary solution to distract you from addressing the tough issue of losing weight and keeping it off.

Instead of jumping on the diet bandwagons, and learning to cope with its highs and lows, eat as outlined in Chapter 6. It sets you up for lasting success by teaching you the right way to think about permanent weight loss.

Unfortunately, this is not headline news. It's not sexy enough to sell millions. But it is effective enough to change your life—and that can be priceless.

To lose weight and keep it off you will need to find a way to eat that allows you to enjoy a healthy and satisfying diet—one that's just for you (for more info, see Chapter 6.) A winning diet gets you active and leaves you feeling full of energy. It addresses underlying emotions that may be at the root of your eating issues. It accomplishes all these points in an organized way, in manageable steps that work for you. It skips the quick fix because that means quick disappointment. (See Chart 5-3)

CHART 5-3

Key Questions to Ask Before You Try Your Next Diet

- Is the diet nutritionally adequate? If an entire category of foods is excluded, such as fat or fruit, chances are you'll experience intense cravings for these foods and may develop true nutritional deficiencies.
- Are there enough calories in the diet? Although everyone thinks less is better, if you eat too few calories, you are more likely to binge. A diet must provide at least as many calories as your body burns, as determined by your resting metabolic rate (Page 111).
- How practical is the plan? Will you always be able to find something to eat regardless of where you are?
- What about cost? If you are required to lay out a sum of money for anything, be careful. Eating right should not cost you more than your average food bill. *Supplements, pills and special foods are rarely necessary in a healthy weight loss plan.*
- How quickly will you lose weight? You should not be promised a weight loss greater than two pounds a week. More than that means you are over-restricting, which ultimately leads to binging. Initial weight loss may be greater than two pounds but it should average out to about 1–2 pounds a week.
- What about your lifestyle? College students rarely eat at the same time everyday. Is the plan flexible enough to accommodate your lifestyle?
- Are you required to think? If you follow a diet pattern but don't look at your eating behavior, you will ultimately get bored with the program and revert to old habits. Permanent weight loss requires behavior change. Nothing is as easy as it seems.
- Do you need to move? Weight loss without a sensible exercise program is hard, if not impossible. Start moving slowly and increase your pace as time goes on.
- Does it sound too good to be true? The bottom line—it probably is.

Beyond Diets: Pills and Surgery

We've all heard the promises of fat burning beverages, pills that rev your metabolism or products that can flush away fat. The late night infomercials and magazine spreads of before and after pictures are convincing—it's hard to not believe they are true. Unfortunately, the diet aids heavily marketed today for weight loss are, for the most part illegal, unsafe or simply ineffective.

Diet drugs, gadgets and potions are nothing new. What is new is the incredible access people have to potentially dangerous products and tools. Couple this accessibility with the increasing incidence and concern over obesity plus the value we place on instant gratification and it's no wonder the diet product industry is where it's at today.

Diet aids are available as prescription drugs, over-the-counter drugs or herbal supplements. The Food and Drug Administration (FDA) regulates prescription drugs and over-the-counter drugs. They have no jurisdiction over herbal supplements. These products are not regulated at all, leaving quality and effectiveness highly variable. All drugs, including those requiring a prescription and those purchased over the counter carry risks. When it comes to weight loss pills, the health consequences of being obese must override the safety risks associated with a drug or supplement in order to warrant its use. *Note: No weight loss drug to date has been the answer to safe and permanent weight loss.*

Diet Aids

Diet aids fall into four categories: **appetite suppressants, metabolism boosters, fat and carb blockers and fat burners.** In each category, you might find some drugs that require a prescription, some that you can buy over-the-counter and some on the shelves at the local health food store. All should carry a "buyer beware" warning.

Appetite Suppressants

Meridia® and phentermine are examples of appetite suppressants available by prescription for those who meet the medical definition of obese: A BMI over 40 usually indicating you are 100 pounds over an ideal weight. (see Chart 6-1) These substances have never been promoted as useful for the person wishing to drop a few pounds, although they often wind up in the medicine cabinets of those people, too.

Meridia and phentermine work by making a person feel full faster. Their effectiveness is modest at best. Weight loss is quickly regained once a person stops taking the drug.

Years ago, over-the-counter weight loss drugs with names like Dexatrim and Acutrim were very popular. They are no longer available at your local pharmacy because they contained the active ingredient phenylpropanolamine (PPA). Significant side affects including heart palpitations and stroke led the FDA to ban PPA from these products. Manufacturers of over-the-counter weight loss aids are no doubt scrambling for a replacement to these products. Buyer beware.

Metabolism Boosters

Metabolism boosters promise weight loss by claiming they help your body burn more calories. Sounds simple. Years ago, the most popular drug used for weight loss was a metabolism booster know as **amphetamine.** Amphetamines are still available, but because of the potential for addiction and abuse, they are rarely prescribed.

Nevertheless, the concept of revving up your metabolism still sells. The most popular over-the-counter metabolism booster was, until recently, **ephedra.** In 2003, the FDA banned its use because of safety concerns, including several deaths associated with its use. Just recently, the case banning ephedra has been challenged. Regardless of the courts decision, the unsupervised use of ephedra carries many risks.

Shortly after ephedra was banned, diet companies began marketing a new product as its replacement. **Synephrine,** marketed as bitter orange, sour orange, green orange and zhi shi, appears to behave like ephedra also. Other popular diet products claim to be "ephedra free". They contain ephedra-like compounds such as ephedrine, norephedrine, pseudoephedrine, methylephedrine and norpseudoephedrine which claim to work similar to ephedra by stimulating the heart and central nervous system and giving the sensation that they are revving your metabolism. Often these products are coupled with caffeine which can also act, to a small degree, as a metabolism stimulant. Using these products can have serious side effects including dramatically increasing your blood pressure and making you feel both jittery and exhausted at the same time. The bottom line is that they do not work for long term weight management.

Caffeine, found in coffee and some sodas, is sometimes categorized as metabolism booster. Anyone who has had too much caffeine may attest to the jolt it delivers. But is it truly a metabolism booster? Probably not. Especially if it comes in the form of a large latte with whipped cream and sugar!

Guarana is another caffeine-containing ingredient found in many diet products. It is marketed as a metabolism booster. While it might make you feel jittery and revved up, it's unlikely that it will actually alter your metabolic rate to any significant extent.

Green tea is a new player in the field of weight loss. It is also linked to a whole host of other health-related issues, such as enhancing immunity and cancer prevention. It is too early to say if all or even some of the claims are true. At this point, it seems unlikely that green tea alone can help you lose weight. It will need to be partnered with a healthy diet and adequate exercise.

Fat and Carb Blockers

Xenical™, a prescription drug, reportedly blocks the body from absorbing fat thereby limiting the number of calories your body can use. Unfortunately, it comes with many unpleasant side effects such as bloating and diarrhea. Like Meridia, once you stop taking Xenical, your body gains back the weight it shed.

Over the counter "fat trappers" are marketed with names such as **chitasan** and their "cousins"—carb blockers. They have never been shown to be helpful in weight loss. While not technically "blockers", some herbal teas claim to help you lose weight, too. These generally contain the ingredient **senna**. Senna may cause increased bowel movements. This does not equate with weight loss. Like all of the above products, it is neither effective or risk free.

Fat Burners

The most popular products claiming to burn away fat contain **chromium** or chromium picolinate. Chromium is needed for regulating blood sugar. However, linking the research on chromium with weight loss is a stretch. The studies do not support this claim, and like most of the other products mentioned thus far, it has risky side effects.

Stomach Stapling and Other Surgeries

Surgery for obesity has come a long way in terms of ease and effectiveness, but it is not the answer for most people wanting to lose weight. Unless you are morbidly obese, meaning you are somewhere in the range of 100 pounds overweight, you are not a candidate for this treatment.

There are several different types of obesity surgeries. Depending on your weight and your medical condition, a "bariatric" surgeon, someone who specializes in treating weight issues, will help you sort through your options. This is an extremely risky, expensive and complicated procedure, regardless of what various Internet sites may say.

It is a life-changing decision with life-threatening potential. Pursuing a surgical approach to treating obesity should be taken very seriously and done with an expert's guidance.

The Bottom Line

Low carb, fat free, high protein . . . regardless of how a diet is dressed up, the bottom line is

- Calories
- The source of one's calories and
- A lifetime commitment to change.

Dieting in the traditional sense never works. It creates a limiting mindset—that of "being good" if you follow the rules and that of "being bad" if you don't.

There are sensible ways to lose weight. For most people, they do not involve trendy diets, drugs or surgery. You can do it enjoyably and successfully if you can get past the hype. Losing weight and keeping it off requires common sense, knowledge and commitment.

Shedding
Excess Weight

Before you get psyched to shed pounds, take time to see if you even need to. You can use a standard height/weight chart (see Chart 6–1) to help determine your desired weight range, or you can use common sense to decide at what weight you feel best and are the healthiest. Your ideal weight should be a range, such as 120 to 130 pounds, not a specific number.

Don't get hung up on numbers alone, though. The scale doesn't tell the whole story. A more important distinction than the number on the scale is how much of your weight is made up of body fat. Weighing more than the charts state as "ideal" isn't bad if you're muscular. However, if your weight is coming from too much fat, it probably is unhealthy and unwanted (see Chart 6–2).

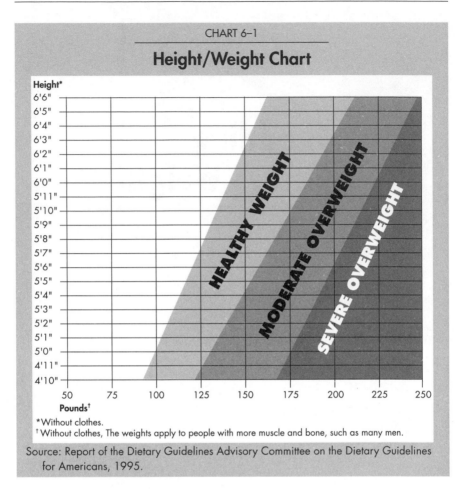

CHART 6–1

Height/Weight Chart

Height*

Source: Report of the Dietary Guidelines Advisory Committee on the Dietary Guidelines for Americans, 1995.

*Without clothes.
†Without clothes, The weights apply to people with more muscle and bone, such as many men.

There are sophisticated methods for determining an accurate body fat measurement, such as skinfold calipers, underwater weighing and bioelectrical impedance. These methods may be available at your school's health service, the physical education department, the local hospital, or a health club. If they're not accessible, you can use a few simple methods to determine whether you're overweight or overfat.

Body Mass Index (BMI)

BMI is a useful index to assess whether you weigh more than you should. A formula is used to determine BMI, but it is presented more simply in Chart 6–3. Closely associated with body fatness, BMI is used by health professionals to assess obesity, and is practical because

CHART 6–2

Are You Too Fat?

Percent of Body Fat

	WOMEN	MEN
Normal	15–25%	10–20%
Overweight	26–29%	21–24%
Obese	>30%	>25%

CHART 6–3

Body Mass Index (BMI)

How to use this chart:

- Locate your height in the left column.
- Follow that row across until you find your weight.
- Look to the number at the top of the column to find your BMI.

BMI   19–24   Healthy weight
BMI   25–29   Overweight
BMI   Above 30 Obese

WEIGHT (IN POUNDS) HEIGHT (IN FEET AND INCHES)

BMI	19	20	21	22	23	24	25	26	27	28	29	30	35	40
4'10"	91	96	100	105	110	115	119	124	129	134	138	143	167	191
4'11"	94	99	104	109	114	119	124	128	133	138	143	148	173	198
5'	97	102	107	112	118	123	128	133	138	143	148	153	179	204
5'1"	100	106	111	116	122	127	132	137	143	148	153	158	185	211
5'2"	104	109	115	120	126	131	136	142	147	153	158	164	191	218
5'3"	107	113	118	124	130	135	141	146	152	158	163	169	197	225
5'4"	110	116	122	128	134	140	145	151	157	163	169	174	204	232
5'5"	114	120	126	132	138	144	150	156	162	168	174	180	210	240
5'6"	118	124	130	136	142	148	155	161	167	173	179	186	216	247
5'7"	121	127	134	140	146	153	159	166	172	178	185	191	223	255
5'8"	125	131	138	144	151	158	164	171	177	184	190	197	230	262
5'9"	128	135	142	149	155	162	169	176	182	189	196	203	236	270
5'10"	132	139	146	153	160	167	174	181	188	195	202	207	243	278
5'11"	136	143	150	157	165	172	179	186	193	200	208	215	250	286
6'	140	147	154	162	169	177	184	191	199	206	213	221	258	294
6'1"	144	151	159	166	174	182	189	197	204	212	219	227	265	302
6'2"	148	155	163	171	179	186	194	202	210	218	225	233	272	311
6'3"	152	160	168	176	184	192	200	208	216	224	232	240	279	319
6'4"	156	164	172	180	189	197	205	213	221	230	238	246	287	328

Source: World Health Organization

it gives a range for ideal weight rather than a specific number. Note to athletes: BMI may not be an accurate tool for you because it does not differentiate the weigh of fat vs. muscle. Many athletes may have a higher than acceptable BMI, but are in fact within an acceptable weight range.

The Eyeball Method

Take a good look in the mirror. Do you see a lot of visible fat, such as "love handles" around your waist, the "extra roll" over the top of your pants, or the infamous "beer belly" around your midsection? Don't compare your physique to stick-thin magazine models; their size is far from reality, and some actually are unhealthy because they're too thin.

The "Pinch an Inch" Test

Using your thumb and forefinger, pinch the skin on the back of your upper arm. This is the spot on your body that is most reliable for predicting overall body fatness. If it's more than an inch thick, you need firming up.

The "I Think My Clothes Shrunk" Test

Do your clothes feel a tad more snug? Having a hard time zipping your jeans? It's possible you have yet to master Laundry 101, but a few extra pounds on your frame may be the culprit. Unless you're really working out and can see a more muscular bod, you've probably gained a few pounds of "real" weight.

If you've determined you need to lose weight, the next step is to decide if you are ready, truly ready, to do it. Your decision to lose weight has to be your own, not your mother's, your boyfriend's, or even your doctor's. Until you are personally motivated to make some changes in how you eat, what you eat, and how physically active you are, no coaxing, joking, or even "caring" by other people will make a difference.

Why Lose Weight?

Studies suggest that being overweight can put you at risk for developing many health problems, such as high blood pressure, diabetes, cancer, and heart disease. Besides reducing future health risks, losing weight has some immediate benefits, including:

You will be better.

If you are significantly overweight, losing weight can give you more energy. Imagine how hard your heart has to work to move an extra 10, 20, or 30 pounds around. Carry a 10, 20, or 30 pound weight in your backpack for an hour and you'll know. It's tiring. Lose weight and you ease your load tremendously; your whole body will signal its appreciation.

If you're involved in sports, losing weight may also help your performance, that's assuming you lose weight safely. The gadget and gimmick approach to weight loss often results in some fat loss, but it also causes loss of muscle and water. The Bottom Line: you lose strength, power, and stamina when you go the gimmick route.

You will look better.

Most people want to lose weight because they want to look better. In our appearance-based society, being overweight often creates an emotional burden. Although losing weight doesn't change your life, if you are overweight, losing will improve your appearance. You'll feel more comfortable physically, and you'll like what you see.

You will feel better.

Even though heart disease, cancer, diabetes, and high blood pressure are not your top concerns right now, sticking to an ideal body weight will make you healthier over the long run. It doesn't take until middle age for obesity to cause these problems. Being overweight can cause high blood pressure at any age. Eighty percent of adults with Type 2 or adult onset diabetes are obese. Obese young adults now account for a growing percentage of people with this type of diabetes. Although it remains unclear how obesity plays a role in the development of cancer, the more weight you carry around at any age, the greater your risk for the disease.

How Much Should You Lose?

Finding a Comfortable Weight Range

Use Chart 6–1 to get an idea of your comfortable weight range. It's tempting to want to reach the weight listed as the lowest amount on the chart. Be realistic. Your goal weight range is one where you feel good, your clothes fit well, and you can eat in a normal non-restrictive way that allows your body to function normally, with plenty of energy and freedom from obsessing about food.

Strive for a healthy, desirable weight, not necessarily what you read about some model weighing or a number you've pulled out of the air because it sounds good. Because we often try to measure up to what we see in the media, we no doubt have a warped concept of a so-called normal body. Keep in mind that most of us won't ever look like super-models. Many hours, much money, and intensive dieting and exercise are spent on trying to achieve and maintain those bodies. It is not a reasonable or ideal body for most young women, so don't try to measure down to those stats.

Even young women at an appropriate weight (read: not rail thin) become caught up in this problem. Seeing everyone dieting and feeling uncomfortable with their bodies, it's a challenge for us to accept a "normal" body. You have to work hard to avoid the dieting trap and stand your ground. Learning to feel good about your weight will free you from a lifetime wasted on body loathing and dieting.

Setting Weight Loss Goals

Next, break your weight loss goal into manageable, achievable steps. It's overwhelming to focus on the big picture alone, such as needing to lose 30 pounds, but it's reasonable to consider shaving five pounds off your frame every month. Studies show that most successful "losers" lose weight in stages. Map out a plan that permits you to lose slowly.

When you reach your first achievable goal, you will have tasted success. Motivation soars. Capitalize on it and dive in for more. Chances are as you reach each new weight goal you'll plateau, or stay at that weight for a while, before you start to lose again. This is a healthy way to let your body and mind adjust to its new size. You may be tempted to restrict your intake even more to get over the plateau. Don't. Instead, be patient and check in by looking carefully at your eating and exercise plan. Are you committed in the same way you were when you started the journey? Hang in there and be vigilant about your plan, but don't shave calories from what allowed you to lose weight initially.

Do the Math

The formula for losing weight is based on the balance between calories taken in and calories burned. If you eat more calories than you expend, you'll gain weight. If you expend more calories than you eat, you'll lose weight. As simple as that sounds, there are many variables that make losing weight complicated.

How much do you eat?

You need an honest assessment of how much you eat (see Chart 6–4). Successfully losing weight doesn't require constant counting, measuring, and recording of each and every morsel of food you put in your mouth, but you do need to be aware of your intake and eating behavior.

It goes without saying that simply recording your intake will change the way you eat. You're less likely to "pick" here and there if you know you'll be writing it down, and most people underestimate the amount of food they eat when they record it.

Once you've recorded your intake, you can estimate how many calories you've eaten using food labels, a calorie-counting book, or internet

---

CHART 6–4

Keeping a Food Diary

This exercise is designed to give you a rough estimate of how much you eat. You can determine your actual calorie intake if you measure everything precisely and then use a calorie-counting book to find out the calories in the food. This is hard work, but you may find it useful. More useful is to get a picture of the little things that add up. Most people can accurately recall what they eat when it is on the plate in front of them but fail to include the fingerful of peanut butter, the crust from your friend's leftover pizza, the French fries you didn't order but ate anyway, and the handful of cereal you grab every time you pass by the cereal box. Use the diary to get a ballpark estimate of the amount of food you eat and to see your eating patterns. To get an accurate recording, record the food as you eat it, not at the end of the day.

---

sites such as www.calorieking.com or www.nutritiondata.com. Come up with a number, then add 200 calories to whatever you've recorded to provide a margin for error.

If you're not into counting calories, become familiar with your portion sizes. Then, reduce your daily intake by one-fourth of what you currently eat.

How much does your body burn?

Next, you need to figure out what your body burns: this is called your **metabolic rate** or **metabolism.** Your resting metabolism (RMR) is the number of calories burned for involuntary functions, like pumping blood through your body, breathing, and just being alive. Your RMR operates 24 hours a day, and accounts for 60 to 75 percent of the total calories you burn. To calculate your RMR, follow the steps outlined in Chart 6–5.

Genetics, body composition, size, and sex all influence your RMR. Just as some people have blue eyes and some have brown, some people are born with a revved-up metabolism; they've been given the genes for a faster metabolism. Others operate at a slower speed.

CHART 6–5

Determining Your Basal Metabolic Rate (BMR)

A. To determine your resting metabolic rate (RMR), the number of calories your body burns at rest:

Women:
1. Begin with a base of 655 calories.   655
2. Multiply your weight (in pounds) x 4.3.   _____
3. Multiply your height (in inches) x 4.7.   _____
4. Add together the totals of 1, 2, and 3.   _____
5. Multiply your age by 4.7.   _____
6. Subtract result of 5 from total of 4.   _____
   This number is your RMR

Men:
1. Begin with a base of 66 calories.   66
2. Multiply your weight (in pounds) x 6.3.   _____
3. Multiply your height (in inches) x 12.7.   _____
4. Add together the totals of 1, 2, and 3.   _____
5. Multiply your age by 6.8.   _____
6. Subtract result of 5 from total of 4.   _____
   This number is your RMR

B. To determine your (BMR), the total number of calories you burn during the day:
1. RMR _____ x 30% (less active days) or
                                                                            = additional calories burned by activity
2. RMR _____ x 40% (more active days)

Add RMR from step A with calories burned from step B. This equals your BMR.

Example:
Julia, a 20 year old young woman who weighs 135 and is 65 inches:

1. Base of   655
2. Weight of 135 x 4.3 =   580.5
3. Height of 65 inches x 4.7   305.5
4. 1+2+3 =   1541
5. Age of 20 x 4.7   94
6. 1541–94 =   **RMR = 1447**

   RMR 1447 x 30%
   434.1 = approximate calories burned on inactive day

BMR = 1447 + 434.1 = 1881.1 calories burned on average day

Body composition influences metabolism because muscle burns more calories than fat. The more muscle you have, the higher your metabolism. Men are naturally more muscular than women, so they tend to have a higher metabolism.

Metabolism is also influenced by size. A long, slender body has more surface than a short, rounded body and requires more calories to maintain normal body temperature. So, long-limbed people will no doubt burn more calories than short people.

Once you know your RMR, you can figure the remaining portion of your total metabolism by adding in the calories you burn by moving your body. While you can't do much to change your sex or genes, exercising and building muscle can change your metabolism. Remember—exercising burns calories, but it also burns body fat and builds muscle, which means that you will burn more calories.

Exercise isn't just the aerobic stuff that takes place at the gym. Simple daily activities such as taking the stairs, walking to class, or vacuuming make the difference between someone who burns a lot versus someone who doesn't.

Creating the Deficit

Once you know how much you eat and how much you burn, you can determine the appropriate calorie intake and amount of food to eat that will allow you to lose one pound. **One pound equals 3500 calories**. Eating 3500 calories above and beyond what you burn makes you gain a pound. So, to lose one pound, you must create a 3500-calorie deficit. By **eliminating 500 calories a day, you could lose 3500 calories or one pound over a week**. You can shave extra food calories (see Chart 6–6) or burn extra calories through favorite activities (see chart 6–7).

It's tempting to try and eliminate as many calories as possible so you'll lose weight rapidly. A pound a week seems unbearably slow! But eating too few calories can be counterproductive. When you severely restrict calories, your body assumes a protective role and tries to conserve energy by lowering metabolism to prevent what it sees as possible starvation. So a diet that is too low in calories can actually sabotage your weight loss efforts by inadvertently lowering your metabolism.

CHART 6–6

Shaving Calories from Your Diet

INSTEAD OF THIS . . .	TRY THIS	CALORIES SAVED
8 oz. 2% milk (120)	8 oz. skim milk (80)	40
1 cup Grape Nuts (416)	1 cup Wheat Chex (150)	266
Ben & Jerry's ice cream (280)	Breyer's ice cream (150)	130
Tuna packed in oil (170)	Tuna packed in water (100)	70
Pizza Hut pepperoni pan pizza (810)	2 slices Plain pizza (480)	330
Big Mac (560)	Cheeseburger (320)	240
Large fries (450)	Small fries (210)	240
6" Meatball sub (420)	6" Turkey sub (290)	130
KFC fried chicken breast (400)	Roast chicken breast, (170)	230
Caesar salad (520)	Caesar salad, no dressing (240)	280
Taco salad (800)	Cheese quesadilla (330)	470
Whole milk Cafe Mocha (400) 16 oz.	Skim milk latte (145) 16 oz.	255

Even when you're trying to lose weight, you need to eat at least as much as your body burns "to stay in business," or to maintain your resting metabolic rate. Since nearly everyone's body at rest burns at least 1200 calories a day, it is rarely recommended for a female to eat fewer than 1200 calories per day and a male fewer than 1500 calories per day.

Eating too little and losing weight too quickly is exactly why dieting fails. If you eat a restrictive diet, you're more likely to binge, and there goes the "perfect" day. Create a weight loss goal to eat as much as you can to lose weight, not as little. You won't restrict food intake and feel deprived, and you won't risk lowering your metabolism. This gives you a much better chance to keep the weight off. If you do it thoughtfully, you won't have to look at those 20 pounds again.

Although weight loss makes sense mathematically, most people don't eat the same way every day, and they don't move their bodies the same amount every day. This makes your rate of weight loss a little less predictable.

People eat for reasons other than hunger, so even if you know exactly how many calories your body burns, and how many calories you eat on any given day, you have to add in other factors. Your personal weight loss plan requires that you explore your eating behavior, the way you think about

CHART 6–7

Sneaking Activity into Your Life

Can't make the time to "workout" regularly? Then sneak activity into your day. Don't underestimate the value of simply moving your body. Take the stairs, walk to and from class, park your car at a space far away or get off the bus a stop early. These all increase your output and make you move more.

Try some of these ideas to fit more movement into an already busy schedule.

1. Bike to class. You will see campus from a different angle.

2. Roller blade or skate board (if permitted) around campus.

3. Instead of meeting a friend for coffee, meet for a walk. Walking with a friend makes it more social and more enjoyable for some.

4. Join an intramural team. Try a sport you've never done before. That's the beauty of intramural sports.

5. Sign up for a P.E. class. Most colleges offer a variety of classes from weight lifting to gymnastics. If you sign up for a class it is a part of your schedule and easier to be committed.

6. Work out at the gym. If you are uncomfortable working out in the gym because you are shy, uncomfortable with your body or just don't know the ins and outs of gyms, call ahead and ask someone to give you a tour. Find out the time of day when the gym is least crowded. After two or three visits, you will feel like a regular.

7. Check out the golf course. Many colleges have access to courses for their students. If you don't know how to play, see if there is a golf class offered your school.

8. Go clubbing. Many schools have clubs that offer all kinds of activities. Try something active like rock climbing, hiking or kayaking.

9. Play frissbee . . . or ultimate frisbee. It's great exercise and so much fun.

10. Walk the dog. Don't have one? Put an ad in the local paper to become a dog walker. Make some extra cash and get in your activity.

OTHER IDEAS TO ADD ACTIVITY TO YOUR LIFE
(these will burn an average of 150 calories)

Washing and waxing a car	45–60 minutes
Walking in the mall	2 hours
Shoveling snow	30 minutes
Raking leaves or sweeping	30 minutes
Playing touch football	30–45 minutes
Cleaning a closet	45–60 minutes

food and how you use food to cope. An eating plan created by someone for you to follow may guide you to desirable food choices. However, only when you change your behavior will your weight loss be permanent.

Playing the Game to Win:
How to eat thin, think thin, get thin, and stay thin

Eating Thin

- Calories count.

  Calories are the bottom line in weight management. It doesn't matter if you eat 100 calories of pretzels or 100 calories of potato chips. A calorie is a calorie.

- All foods fit, theoretically.

  You should learn to eat all the foods you enjoy in reasonable amounts. Cookies, candy, and chips are foods we eat because they taste good, not because we need them. Use them at the end of a meal, not when you're very hungry and will overeat. Start by including these foods in portion-controlled servings. Eat an ice cream sandwich rather than keeping a carton of ice cream or frozen yogurt in the freezer. Add a single-serving bag of chips to your lunch instead of eating the jumbo bag as a late-night snack.

- Don't eat anything you don't like, even if you know it is good for you.

  Calories are too precious to waste on things you **should** eat. Sometimes we're driven by guilt to eat so-called good foods. Then we eat what we really want. If your diet is satisfying and includes food that tastes good to you, eventually you'll eat less. Although you can't abandon the basic nutrition principles outlined in Chapter 1, your diet doesn't need to be perfect to be healthy.

- Eliminate grazing.

  Grazing is the downfall of any college student. Handfuls of food, even "healthy" food, will add up the calories but not satisfy. (see Chart 6–8) Grazers are often afraid to eat something big, so they

CHART 6–8

Grazing by the Handful

FOOD	HANDFULS	CALORIES
Pirates Booty	2	100
Frosted cereal	2	250
Pretzel rings	2	220
Tostitos	2	300
Granola	2	330
Trail mix	2	360
Almonds	2	680

would rather nibble their way through the day. The problem is, the calories add up way too quickly. Try to work real mealtimes and satisfying snacks into your schedule, even if you eat them while sitting in class (see Chart 6–9).

- Learn to love water.

  If you have your own refrigerator, keep a pitcher of water in it. Start each meal with a glass of water. It will allow you to think about the food you eat, and it's great for your complexion.

- Don't drink your calories.

  If you fill up on soda and juice, you won't satisfy hunger or thirst, yet you'll consume a lot of calories (see Chart 6–10). Learn to drink water to satisfy your thirst and save soda and juice for special occasions. Diet sodas don't satisfy thirst or hunger either. Although the price of bottled water is sometimes prohibitive, carry a bottle with you and refill it.

- Start the day strong.

  Breakfast jump-starts your metabolism and gets you going. Some people skip breakfast because they see that as an easy way to shave calories off the day. However, most of these same people end up overcompensating for the calories they missed by overeating later in the day.

CHART 6–9

Satisfying Snack Foods to Beat Grazing

Snacking should bridge the gap between meals. Consider snacks mini meals. Sit down, put the food on a plate or in a bowl, and pay attention to what you are eating rather than grabbing from a box until it's empty. The snacks listed below range from very filling to just enough to get you through an hour or two until dinner.

- Instant hot cereal packages
- Soup: canned soup including vegetable, tomato, chicken noodle; dehydrated soup including Knorr's, Fantastic Food, Nile Spice, Far East (avoid ramen noodles unless they're baked)
- English muffin or 2 slices of toast spread with margarine, butter, apple butter, or peanut butter (about 1 Tbsp.)
- 2 hard-boiled eggs
- Carton of yogurt and toast
- 1 oz. (small box) cereal and skim milk
- Breakfast bar and skim milk
- Skim milk latte
- Fruit and cottage cheese
- Flour tortilla filled with salsa and 2 Tbsp. of grated cheese, cottage cheese mixed with applesauce, 1 Tbsp. hummus, or mashed bean spread
- Peanut butter on an English muffin
- Steamed edamame and tea
- String cheese and a pear

- Balance your choices.

  A healthy diet includes protein, fat, and carbohydrate. Many popular diets are based on eliminating one of these three nutrients. This creates a nutritional imbalance that ultimately results in cravings, nutritional deficiency, or just not sticking with the program.

- Check in to your eating cues.

  If people ate only to satisfy hunger and ate just enough to feel satisfied but not stuffed, chances are the dieting industry would go bust. However, hunger is only one of many reasons why people eat. Learn to check into your feelings of hunger, those cues that should motivate you to eat. Your stomach may grumble or you

CHART 6–10

Drinking Your Calories

FOOD	SERVING	CALORIES
Soda	12 oz. can	140
Orange juice	8 oz.	110
Grapefruit juice	8 oz.	100
Grape juice	8 oz.	155
Apple juice	8 oz.	120
Tomato juice	6 oz.	35
Frappucino	grande	260
Commercial drinks (Snapple, Fresh Samantha, etc.)	12 oz.	110–350
Smoothies	12 oz.	220–400
Iced tea	12 oz.	110–160
Skim milk	8 oz.	80
2% milk	8 oz.	120
Whole milk	8 oz.	150
Water	8 oz.	0

may even have a slight headache if you are too hungry. Check out the hunger/fullness scale in Chart 6–11. Ask yourself each time you eat, "Am I hungry?" If you aren't physically hungry but do have an urge to eat, ask yourself what it is that you really need. Are you bored, stressed, sad? Learn to label your feelings and respond to them with something other than food.

• Stop eating when you are full.

To understand fullness, you need to pay attention to what you are eating and to eat it slowly. By eating slowly rather than inhaling your food, you're more likely to receive the signals your body gives you when you're full. Eating rapidly usually leads to overeating; you bypass full and head toward stuffed. Certain foods, especially those high in fiber, may make you feel full.

CHART 6–11

Hunger Scale

Starving and Beyond. ← 0

You are so hungry you want to order everything on the menu. ← 1

Everything on a menu begins to look good. You may be very preoccupied with your hunger. ← 2

You are hungry and the urge to eat is strong. ← 3

A little hungry. You can wait to eat, but you know you will be getting hungry soon. ← 4

Neutral. Not hungry. Not full. ← 5

No longer hungry, You sense food in your belly, but you could definitely eat more. ← 6

Hunger is definitely gone. Stop here, and you may not feel hungry for 3-4 hours. ← 7

Not uncomfortable, but definitely have eaten a belly full. ← 8

Moving into uncomfortable ← 9

"Thanksgiving full." Very uncomfortable, maybe even painful ← 10

This is a rough guideline to introduce you to the Hunger/Satiety Scale. Use these descriptions loosely, hunger and satiety are very subjective experiences. Refine these descriptions by discussing them with your counselor.

To use this scale rate your hunger level before you eat and again and when you are finished eating. It could look like a graph*. If you do this each time you eat, you will become more familiar with your eating patterns, especially if you discuss it with another person. Move away from using your head to decide your eating patterns and towards listening to your body.

*Example—the graph represents:

A meal where you eat from 3 to 7.

A meal where you began eating when you were not hungry, eating from a 6 to 8.

Eating from 2 to 8, from very hungry to uncomfortably full.

Reprinted with permission of author, Karin Kratina in *Moving Away From Diets*. 1996. Lake Dallas, TX: Helm Seminars Publishing.

Thinking Thin

- Forget black and white thinking.

  People fail at long-term weight loss when they think in absolutes. The real world of eating has many shades of gray. **Sometimes** you can eat chocolate, **many** days you'll exercise, **occasionally** you'll want to snack late at night, and **sporadically** you sleep through breakfast.

- Perfection doesn't count.

  You'll always face challenging eating situations. You may over-eat or you may not have an opportunity to exercise, and, as a result, you may gain weight. The key to successful weight loss is to regroup. Don't let one episode of backsliding signal the beginning of the end. Instead, consider it part of the learning curve, and acknowledge the experience as bringing you a step closer to being a more experienced, healthy eater.

- Learn to eat, not to diet.

  Swear off dieting. When you "go on a diet," you will then go off a diet. Dieting is restricting, and restriction never works.

- Face the food.

  If you can't face your food—literally—you shouldn't eat it. Absent-mindedly grabbing popcorn from a bowl while you watch TV or study is not a satisfying way to eat. You tend to eat considerably more than what you need, and you may never really feel full. Eat slowly and enjoy every bite.

Getting Thin

- Move it to lose it.

  Exercising to lose weight should include something aerobic such as biking, running, brisk walking, or swimming done for 35–45 minutes, four to five times a week. You can also get your exercise by doing something more moderate, but for a longer time such as walking, playing golf or even shopping.

- Manage cravings.

Cravings are an intense desire for a particular food and are usually unrelated to hunger. If you seriously restrict how much you eat, you're more likely to experience cravings. Try and include favorite foods in reasonable amounts. For instance, if cookies are your craving, eat them with a meal instead of hoarding them in your dorm room or pantry and then bingeing on them (see Chart 6–12).

- Pick a pattern.

Eating every three to five hours works best for most people. If you go through the day without eating and then begin eating late in the day, your eating is more likely to be out of control.

CHART 6–12

Managing Cravings

Cravings . . . an intense desire to eat a specific food usually unrelated to hunger. They spell doom for any dieter. But they're normal and they don't have to "do you in." Take these steps to manage your cravings rather than pretending you can override and ultimately forget them.

- Set a timer before you start eating. Make eating anything a conscious act. Have a list of things you can do instead of eating. If you have to create the list as the craving strikes, you're sunk. Cravings dominate, so be prepared with the list (see Chart 4–4).

- Select a reasonable amount of food. One cookie isn't reasonable and six may seem like too many. But if you actually eat four you'll feel successful.

- Don't try to fool yourself by eating the so-called good foods first. If you start out craving chocolate, baby carrots are not likely to satisfy you. Instead of working your way around the craving, start with the food you want. Ask yourself what it is you're craving specifically: salt, sugar, fat, warmth, cold, crunchy.

- Sit down and face the food. Standing and eating lets you pretend it didn't happen and doesn't count.

- Make eating an experience in and of itself.

  If you eat standing up or driving in your car, you won't focus on what you've consumed. You'll feel less satisfied and more inclined to keep eating.

- Be the last one finished.

  Whether you're eating a grilled chicken breast or an ice cream sundae, learn to eat slowly and savor each bite. If you're a fast eater, challenge yourself to make the meal last a certain amount of time.

Staying Thin

- Set reasonable goals.

  Many diets fail because you've established unrealistic goals. Although your ultimate objective is to lose weight, you'll need to change many behaviors to get there. Pick small steps related to your diet and exercise habits. Set one or two useful goals at a time and be sure they're specific and forgiving. For instance, "exercise more" is not specific. "Go to the gym every day" is not attainable and requires an ideal situation. Instead, set a goal by saying, " I'll go to the gym four days this week."

- Eat purposefully.

  Eating well takes practice. You need to be aware of each eating episode. By doing so, you'll decrease impulsive eating, the kind that often leads to overeating. You can do this more easily if you establish a habit of asking yourself, before you grab a handful of anything, "Am I hungry?" or "Do I want this or do I need this?" Although you may sometimes decide that indeed you don't need the food, you merely want it, the act of eating the food will then be a conscious decision, and you may be more apt to eat less.

- Have a support network.

  Make a list of things you can do instead of eating. Keep the list front and center, because if you're tempted to do some non-hunger eating, it's often hard to break free and do something different. We often resort to food because it's a comfortable habit. When the going gets tough, know that you can call a friend, call home, e-mail your buddy, take a bath, take a walk, write your feelings in a journal, or just scream and shout.

- Find time to exercise.

  Here's the truth: After a certain age, and you're approaching it, you can maintain weight loss only if you add some exercise to your routine. You don't need to "go for the burn." If exercise hurts, you're less likely to keep it up. If walking feels better than running, take a walk. If you can, enlist a friend. Make your exercise time a social time as well. At the very least, put on a tape and let your brain relax; you'll feel refreshed afterward.

- Know thyself.

  You may never be able to eat some foods with the utmost control—in these situations, it's best to avoid unlimited access to those foods. For instance, keeping a gallon of ice cream in your freezer may be too tempting, but taking yourself out for a cone three times a week might curb your craving. Although it may seem less economical to do it this way, it's a drop in the bucket compared with what most people spend on dieting gimmicks that don't work.

- Monitor your progress.

  This doesn't mean stepping on a scale three times a day—which would be a bit obsessive and counterproductive as well. But you could put on a pair of pants once a week and see how they fit, or measure the increasing distance you're now able to run or walk, or even evaluate periodically what you're choosing to eat to see how it has changed. Reward yourself often. Rewards can be tangible (a new CD, nail polish, or magazine) or intangible (a bath, a nap, or a long walk alone).

Online diet resources

www.weightwatchers.com
www.ediets.com

Books

Fletcher, A. 2003. *Thin for Life*. Boston: Houghton Mifflin

Kirby, J., 2004. *Dieting for Dummies*, 2nd edition. Indianapolis: Wiley Publishing

Rolls, B., 2005. *The Volumetrics Eating Plan*. New York: Harper Collins.

Tribole, E., and E. Resch, 2003. *Intuitive Eating*: A Revolutionary Program That Works. New York: St. Martin's Press.

7

Eating Disorders On Campus

College students lament that everyone seems consumed by food. While this is an exaggeration, students are either dieting and not eating, or, at the opposite extreme, bingeing and gorging on food. The number of college students, primarily women, who are obsessed with what they eat is growing dramatically. On any given day, one out of every two students is on a diet, and an estimated 20–30 percent of students have some type of serious eating disorder. A recent survey of college-age women found that nearly 75 percent classify themselves as overweight, even though most are within a normal weight range. Take the quiz in Chart 7–1 to determine whether you have an eating problem.

Unfortunately, women's dissatisfaction with their bodies gets plenty of reinforcement. The constant self-loathing that precedes and follows

---

CHART 7–1

Do You Have an Eating Problem?

Do you have a normal relationship with food or are you ruled by dieting? To find out, answer these questions:

1. Do you diet often?
2. Do you ever change your plans because you are concerned about the food available?
3. Do you weigh yourself more than once a day?
4. Does the number on the scale affect your day?
5. Do you prefer to eat alone?
6. Are you concerned about what people see you eating?
7. Are you preoccupied with food?
8. Do you feel guilty if you overeat?
9. Do you push yourself to exercise if you've overeaten?
10. Are you troubled if someone tampers with "your" food?
11. Do you have any rituals related to your eating?
12. Do you eat without tasting?

Answering yes to many of these questions may signal an eating problem.

---

a diet is a common dialect among girls, including some as young as age six. By the time they get to college, they've found plenty of kindred spirits. In fact, one hears stories of group bingeing and purging sessions. In some instances, anorexics are held in high regard by their peers because they have achieved "the goal"—being ultra-thin. Being a normal weight and liking that body is hard when you see ultra-thin girls parading around in what's considered to be the most fashionable clothing, designed for the anorexic body.

There hasn't always been hysteria over food and weight. This generation, yours, is the first to be brought up by parents who have embraced dieting as a way of life. Weight Watchers, the pioneer of commercial weight loss programs, was born in the 1960s, just about the same time the envied, voluptuous Marilyn Monroe body type was replaced by Twiggy, the first androgynous-looking, stick-thin glamour girl. Flip through any fashion magazine, and you'll see that her legacy lives on.

There are pages upon pages of ultra-thin models who not only look starved, but literally may be. Many cover girls would easily meet the diagnostic criteria for anorexia, and malnutrition.

Dieting is driven by waif-like images that the fashion and media industries hold up as the ideal. What you may not know is how often and to what extent the photographs of these picture-perfect models have been retouched. These models may have had surgical modifications, too, such as implants, nips, tucks, and enhancements, to get "the look." Some models have gone so far as to have their bottom ribs removed to make their stomachs appear more concave. If you consider these the standard to measure yourself against, you are destined to be frustrated, depressed, and constantly dissatisfied with your most important asset—your body. (See Chart 7–2.)

Eating Disorders

One in ten women has a diagnosed eating disorder and approximately eight in ten float in and out of what's termed disordered eating. While eating disorders must meet specific criteria, "disordered eating" is a pattern of behaviors. Sometimes you overeat, sometimes you diet, but you rarely approach food comfortably and you have a negative attitude about weight and your body. Disordered eating can be the prelude to developing a more life-threatening disorder such as anorexia nervosa, or it can remain a chronic condition you learn to tolerate. But it ultimately drives a wedge between you and the happiness you could otherwise achieve. (See Chart 7–3.)

America's preoccupation with dieting and the quest for trimness parallels the recent increase in diagnosed cases of eating disorders. However, eating disorders are not about dieting or being slim. In fact, the term "eating disorder" is a misnomer; it implies that the problem is rooted in eating, and the solution is simply to "fix" the eating problem.

The roots of an eating disorder are complex. They are the result of psychological problems having to do with self-esteem, control, conflict resolution, and power. Dieting behavior is simply in almost every instance, a symptom of a much larger problem.

CHART 7–2

Building a Better Body Image

Body image can be defined as:
- What you see when you look in the mirror or when you picture yourself in your mind.
- How you think and feel about your body, specifically your height, shape, and weight.
- How you feel **in** your body, which is reflected in how you control your body as you move.

A negative body image is when:
- You perceive parts of your body unlike they really are. Negative attributes are usually given to a specific area such as your hips, thighs, butt, cheeks, or stomach.
- You see your body as too big, regardless of what you weigh.
- You believe that other people are attractive, but you're not.
- You see your body size or shape as a sign of personal failure.
- People describe your size and shape differently from how you do.
- You feel embarrassed, self-conscious, and anxious about your body.
- You feel fatter on days when you're upset and thinner on days when you feel good.

Positive body image is when:
- You see your body as it really is.
- You accept and appreciate your body shape and understand that a person's physical appearance has little to do with his or her value as a person.
- You don't spend an unreasonable amount of time worrying about the food you eat or what the scale says.
- You feel comfortable in your body.

Two exercises to determine whether perception is reality:
1. Using an old bed sheet or large piece of paper, draw an outline of your body. Then, lie down on the sheet or paper and, using a different color marker, have someone actually trace your body. Compare the two. Is your traced body similar in size and shape to the outline you drew? If it is, you have an accurate perception of your body.
2. Stand in front of a mirror. Close your eyes and hold your arms apart to show the width of your body at its widest part. Open your eyes and compare your outstretched arms to what you see.

CHART 7–3

The Eating Issues & Body Image Continuum

This continuum represents the range of eating behaviors and attitudes towards food and body image. Most healthy people function in the two categories on the far left that reflect high self-esteem and physical health: "Concerned Well," and "Not An Issue." However, individuals can move from one category to another depending on changes that occur in their self-esteem and attitudes toward food and body image. An individual can be in one category for food and another category for body image. Also, an individual can exhibit some, but not all, characteristics within a category.

FOOD IS NOT AN ISSUE / BODY OWNERSHIP	CONCERNED WELL / BODY ACCEPTANCE	FOOD PREOCCUPIED/OBSESSED / BODY PREOCCUPIED/OBSESSED	DISRUPTIVE EATING PATTERNS / DISTORTED BODY IMAGE	EATING DISORDERED / BODY HATE/DISASSOCIATION
I am not concerned about what others think regarding what and how much I eat. I feel no guilt or shame no matter how much I eat or what I eat. Food is an important part of my life, but only occupies a small part of my time. I trust my body to tell me what and how much to eat.	I pay attention to what I eat in order to maintain a healthy body. I may weigh more than the "thin ideal," but I enjoy eating and balance my pleasure with eating with my concern for a healthy body. I am moderate and flexible in goals for eating well. I try to follow nutrition guidelines and eat in a balanced way.	I think about food a lot and regularly watch what I eat. It's hard for me to enjoy eating with others. I have tried dieting, excluding certain foods, or counting calories to lose weight. I feel ashamed when I eat more than others or more than what I feel I should be eating. I am afraid of getting fat. I wish I could change how much I want to eat and what I am hungry for.	I have tried diet pills, supplements, laxatives, vomiting or extra time exercising in order to lose or maintain my weight. I have fasted or avoided eating for long periods of time in order to lose or maintain my weight. I feel strong when I can restrict how much I eat. Eating more than I wanted to makes me feel out of control.	I regularly exercise, vomit, use diet pills, supplements or laxatives to get rid of the food or calories. My friends/family tell me I am too thin. I am terrified of eating fat. When I let myself eat, I have a hard time controlling the amount of food I eat. I am afraid to eat in front of others.
I feel good about my body and what it can do. My body is beautiful to me. I reject society's narrow definition of thinness as the only ideal body shape; I believe that healthy and beautiful bodies come in all shapes and sizes. I know that the significant others in my life will always find me attractive. I trust my body to find the weight it needs to be at so I can move and feel confident of my physical body.	I base my body image equally on social norms and my own self-concept. I pay attention to my body and my appearance because it is important to me, but it only occupies a small part of my day. I nourish my body so it has the strength and energy to achieve my physical goals. I am able to assert myself and maintain a healthy body without losing my self-esteem.	I spend a significant amount of time viewing my body in the mirror. I spend a significant amount of time comparing my body to others. I have many days when I feel fat. I am preoccupied with my body. I accept society's thin ideal body shape and size as the best body shape and size. I'd be more attractive if I was thinner, more muscular, etc...	I spend a significant amount of time exercising and dieting to change my body. I believe that my body shape and size keeps me from dating or finding someone who will treat me the way I want to be treated. I have considered changing or have changed my body shape and size through surgical means, so I can accept myself. I wish I could change the way I look in the mirror.	I often feel separated and distant from my body—as if it belongs to someone else. I hate my body and I often isolate myself from others. I don't see anything positive or even neutral about my body shape and size. I don't believe others when they tell me I look OK. I hate the way I look in the mirror.

Used with permission. (Smiley/King/Avey, 1996, University of Arizona)

The Start of a Problem

An eating disorder often begins as an ordinary attempt to lose weight. You lose weight, get compliments on your appearance, and all of a sudden you feel a sense of control, power, and superiority. You've succeeded where others have not. Your sense of identity, security, and control become tied to your ability to lose weight. No one starts dieting with the idea of developing an eating disorder. And, obviously everyone who diets is not at risk for developing one. Yet, most people diagnosed with an eating disorder admit to dieting at some point in their lives. Chronic dieting, along with a society that reveres the hollow-cheeked look, serves as a perfect springboard for a vulnerable young adult to develop an eating disorder.

Anorexia

Anorexia nervosa is a psychological disorder in which you purposely lose weight as a result of dieting, but the dieting gets out of control. New research shows that genetics plays a role in susceptibility to this illness, but its exact role isn't yet clear. What has emerged, through various studies, are characteristics of people with eating disorders. They include:

- They are often thought of as compliant kids, ones who are a bit shy, good students, often perfectionists.
- They are eager to please, but they haven't figured out how to please themselves. Their success at dieting fills this void in their life.
- They get a sense of power from their weight loss and satisfaction from controlling what and how much they eat. The control they have over food and over their bodies becomes their identity. It is hard to relinquish that identity, even though they are becoming hazardously thin. They never consider themselves thin enough. **Denial is a hallmark characteristic of anorexia nervosa.**

Anorexia is not only about looking thin, it's a mindset as well. The effort and energy it takes to be and stay bone-thin is all-consuming.

You spend every waking minute thinking about food, body size, and weight. You become so preoccupied with food that it interferes with many other aspects of your life. What kind of food will be at the party? Can I exercise if I go away for the weekend? Where will I weigh myself? All are common, self-absorbed thoughts.

These struggles with anorexia make a person irritable, unable to concentrate, and, quite frankly, a drag to be around. It becomes easier and less confrontational for anorexics to spend time alone, so people with anorexia often isolate themselves. Depression ensues. You become so self-absorbed with this disease, it's difficult to think about anything else but yourself. School, friends, and relationships are neglected.

Without food to fuel the brain and with most of one's energy channeled toward staying thin, social relationships evaporate. The number on the scale never seems acceptable. A lower weight is always the goal,

CHART 7–4

Signs and Symptoms of Anorexia Nervosa

- Weight loss leading to a body weight of 85 percent of what's considered acceptable
- Intense fear of being "fat" or gaining weight
- Disturbed body image; feels fat in spite of extremely low weight
- Frequent weighing
- Denies hunger
- Develops ritualistic eating habits, such as cutting food into tiny pieces, eating alone, and dragging out meals
- Loss of menstrual period
- Excessive exercise
- Rigid about food and meals
- Creates list of foods not liked or avoided for "legitimate" reasons—such as being a vegetarian or being lactose intolerant
- Perfectionist
- Preoccupied with food: cooks and prepares food for others, may be involved in food-related work, watches food shows, and reads recipes constantly
- Increased sensitivity to cold
- Refuses to admit eating patterns are abnormal
- Withdraws socially

until ultimately a person with anorexia becomes miserable and very sick (see Chart 7–4).

Bulimia

In sharp contrast to anorexia is bulimia, which is more widespread than anorexia. It is characterized by bingeing, or eating a large amount of food (anywhere from 1000 to 50,000 calories) in a short period of time. The bulimic then purges to get rid of the food. Purging takes the form of vomiting, laxative abuse, diuretic abuse, and even excessive exercising (see Chart 7–5). Unless you've actually witnessed someone purging, it's much harder to identify people with bulimia than those with anorexia. Most are of normal weight, some are even overweight.

Like anorexia, bulimia is a psychosocial problem. Self-deprecating thoughts, such as an inability to measure up and a relentless sense of body loathing, characterize this illness too. While anorexics thrive on order, people with bulimia generally have a more chaotic lifestyle. They turn to bingeing and purging as a way to deal with stress or conflict, or as a way to gain control over a seemingly out-of-control life. People with bulimia are well aware of the dangers of their illness, but are too ashamed or embarrassed to ask for help.

For many bulimics, purging feels necessary and good. It's a way of regaining control after gorging on an excessive amount of food. The sense of "cleansing" felt after using laxatives or throwing up is seductive. It becomes the antidote to the binge. Before long, a person with bulimia is planning her days around when or where she can purge.

Bulimia sends the body mixed signals: here's some food, now it's gone. The result is that the body is in a constant state of hunger, and the urge to eat/binge becomes overwhelming. Overeating is inevitable, making the purge seem necessary. A cycle develops, and it becomes difficult to find a way out. More often than not, the person with bulimia gains weight.

If you've just polished off a sleeve of cookies, you're not necessarily considered bulimic. Everyone binges on occasion. Purging after a binge, however, is the defining characteristic of bulimia. And although you may have given a passing thought to running off all of those cookies or dashing to the toilet for relief, for the person with bulimia, purging is

---

CHART 7–5

Exercise Bulimia

Obsessed With Exercise
by Karin Kratina, M.A., R.D., L.D.

In this age of fitness, many of us admire those dedicated people who seem to be able to make it to the gym no matter what. Rain, snow, sleet, cancelled dates, lost sleep, whatever it takes, they get their workout each day. They appear to be in great shape, highly motivated and apparently very healthy. But maybe not. Looks can be deceiving.

Rather than being fitness buffs, they may have crossed over the line to fanaticism. They continue to run, lift and bike, ignoring torn ligaments, fractured bones, loss of menstrual cycle and other health problems.

Many of us worry about weight gain and will diet or wish we were a little thinner. We might exercise occasionally to get back in shape (or maybe exercise everyday for the first two weeks until we get bored). We may exercise so we can eat a little more and maintain our weight. We consider workouts important, but we don't feel a compulsive drive to complete them.

When that compulsiveness is present-when a person's life becomes centered around food, weight and exercise and when significant decisions are based on how much we have eaten, on what the scale says, or on how much exercise we can fit in-an eating disorder may exist.

Although exercise doesn't always correlate with an eating disorder, vigorous exercise to prevent weight gain is one of the diagnostic criteria for bulimia.

Exercise bulimics and anorexics are difficult to identify. When a person uses exercise as a method of purging, he/she may also get a lot of positive reinforcement. People are usually very impressed with their discipline; most even wish they could keep their own fitness program going. The person who uses exercise to keep his/her weight down and/or to purge doesn't have to keep their strategy a secret. They actually brag about it.

Exercise can ease the stress of a hard day at work, the pain of lost love, and even the embarrassment of forgetting someone's name. This is okay, if the feelings are also dealt with effectively. But, that is not always the case. Exercise can function to distract feelings and ease depression while the issues that need to be confronted are pushed out of the way. For an exercise bulimic or anorectic, the mere thought of missing a workout causes anxiety. To actually stop working out causes withdrawal symptoms such as confusion, irritability, anxiety, depression and lack of energy as well as decreased self-confidence and self-esteem. Some people with eating disorders continue to exercise while injured and will organize their activities around exercise. Significant decisions (from interviewing for a job to accepting a date) are based on how much exercise can be squeezed in. Family, friends and even careers can be ignored. These people need to exercise to be able to function from day to day.

Some professionals believe that all people who exercise regularly are addicted to some degree. One popular theory, as yet unproven, is that the compulsive exercisers become hooked on hormones called endorphins. These natural pain killers are released into the bloodstream during strenuous exercise and have been thought to cause the feelings of well-being often accompanied by excessive exercise. Since no one has actually proven endorphins to be psychologically addictive, it may be that this "runner's high" is caused by the release of stress and tension built up during the day.

Exercise addicts develop a powerful sense of control. They feel invincible in an otherwise chaotic life. Many of the people who are addicted set goals that they believe will earn them respect. Once these goals are achieved, however, they convince themselves they can do better and raise their goals. If the goals are achieved or removed, the drive to work out would no longer exist, forcing them to face the emptiness they have exercised to avoid.

When caught in the compulsion, eating disordered people must first acknowledge that a problem exists and move forward to learn how to redefine the purpose of exercise in their lives. Some may need to work with a therapist to find out what issues are locking them into this compulsion. A therapist can help identify how they currently benefit psychologically from the excessive exercise in terms of self-esteem and stress management. The therapist can also help them explore other activities that might offer similar rewards.

With some effort and support, people can learn the difference between healthy and unhealthy exercise and working out because they want to, not because they have to. They can begin to regard working out as something to be done for health and fun, not escape.

Kratina, K. "Obsessed With Exercise." Professional Counselor. 1991; 5(6): 19. Reprinted with permission of Karin Kratina addictive. It becomes difficult for them to cope unless they know where and when they will be able to purge (see Chart 7–6).

Anorexia and bulimia can often be present at the same time. An anorexic may consider a "binge" something consumed outside of her carefully controlled portion of food, even if it's merely an extra two cookies. She then purges by overexercising, using a laxative, or throwing up to eliminate the extra 100 calories. This is an extremely serious situation.

CHART 7–6

Signs and Symptoms of Bulimia

- Preoccupation with food, weight, and appearance
- Eats large volumes of food and then "gets rid" of it by vomiting, fasting, exercising, or taking laxatives
- Makes excuses to go to the bathroom after eating
- Usually near a normal weight, but with weight fluctuations
- Experiences mood swings and depression
- Dental problems
- Stomach and digestive problems—such as bloating, constipation, diarrhea
- Scratched or scarred knuckles from scraping against teeth to induce vomiting
- Irritation of the esophagus and throat
- Low self-esteem
- Realization that eating pattern is abnormal
- Constant feelings of hunger
- Irregular menstrual periods
- Lightheadedness and headaches

Binge Eating

Only recently has binge eating been considered an eating disorder. It is characterized by the consumption of large quantities of food. Unlike bulimia, victims do not purge. The binge is followed instead by feelings of guilt and shame. If you've ever overindulged, you may empathize with this scene, but under normal eating conditions, you get over the splurge and get on with life. However, many people with this disorder are depressed. People who binge don't tend to rebound from their post-binge funk (see Chart 7–7).

CHART 7–7

Signs and Symptoms of Binge Eating Disorder

- Weight gain or obesity
- Stomach and digestive problems
- Eats quickly
- Eats when not physically hungry or binge eats
- Preoccupied with eating, dieting, and weight
- Frequent dieting, without losing weight
- Eats to escape problems and emotions
- Eats "normally" or "diets" with others, then eats large amounts of food when alone
- Eats to the point of feeling uncomfortably full
- Feels guilty or depressed after a binge
- Low self-esteem
- Realizes that eating pattern is abnormal

Health Problems Caused by Eating Disorders

Untreated eating disorders can cause devastating and irreversible changes to your body. At worst, they can be fatal. Approximately 6 to 10 percent of eating-disordered victims die from the disease.

Once the amount of fat on a woman's body dips below 10 percent, she may stop menstruating. The prolonged absence of a menstrual period can cause permanent bone loss, which, in turn, can result in early onset of osteoporosis-thinning and weakening of the bones. It's ironic that young women so focused on a perfect body can unintentionally cause irreversible changes that mirror those of a hunchbacked 80-year-old woman. The lack of a menstrual period, a low-fat intake, and insufficient body fat, may also adversely influence fertility and lower the chance of having a baby sometime in the future.

The problems caused by bulimia are just as serious. Unnaturally regurgitating the contents of your stomach, including its acids, can erode the enamel on your teeth and cause ulcers in your esophagus. Excessive purging of any kind also puts you at risk for developing life-threatening heart and kidney problems. The sooner you get help, the greater your chances for limiting permanent physical and emotional damage.

Helping Someone You Know with an Eating Disorder

Helping someone with an eating disorder is challenging, particularly when that person is in denial which is often the case (see Chart 7–8). You shouldn't try to function as a therapist, doctor, or nutritionist. However, you can confront your friend and assist her in finding professional help. If this feels intrusive, consult your dorm's resident advisor, a college counselor, the health service, or even your friend's parents. As eating disorders have become more prevalent, support services and treatment resources on campuses have become more accessible.

If You Have a Problem

Admitting that you have an eating disorder is difficult, and denial prevents many from seeking help. Because there is an addictive

---

CHART 7–8

How to Help a Friend with an Eating Disorder

- Choose a time and place to talk away from distractions and other interruptions.
- Don't be judgmental. Describe specific observations that have given you concern, rather than judging actions—such as not eating enough, exercising too much, or being too thin.
- Be a good listener, but don't promise to keep serious information confidential. Caring for your friend doesn't mean you should be manipulated because you're "the only one who understands."
- Don't assume the role of therapist or nutritionist. Eating disorders are a serious problem. Don't label the problem as such, but encourage your friend to seek professional help. Do the legwork for her if necessary to find help, and offer to accompany her to the appointment if you're comfortable doing that.
- Don't oversimplify the problem by saying, "All you have to do is eat." This is a complex problem, and dwelling on weight, eating, and appearance won't solve it.
- Don't engage in a battle, but don't ignore the problem. If your friend denies having a problem, don't be deceived by her excuses. Instead, state the facts: you're concerned, you've observed a situation that appears unhealthy, and you think this needs to be checked out by a professional.

component to the illness, it can be difficult to overcome on your own. Often people struggling with a disorder feel trapped. Being away from home can compound the problem, since you're on your own with little support. It can make being sick a scary and lonely experience. If you think you have an eating disorder, or if friends are expressing concern over your appearance, talk with an expert.

Treatment

Treating an eating disorder is a "team" effort that includes a doctor, a therapist, a nutritionist, you, and often your family. It doesn't matter who you consult first, just be sure that he or she is skilled in working with eating disorders.

- A therapist will help you understand the real problems that triggered the disease.
- A doctor will evaluate the extent of physical damage and work with you to correct it. He or she will monitor your weight, blood pressure, and other vital signs, and prescribe medication if needed.
- Many eating-disordered victims are self-professed nutrition experts, but they've lost sight of what constitutes normal eating. A nutritionist can help you determine an ideal weight range and work with you to develop healthy eating habits.

Because the process is long and arduous, it may help to take a leave from school while you recover. Recovering can be a full-time undertaking, but if you are committed to getting better, you can. Relapse is always a concern, but with treatment you'll learn the warning signs for relapse and you'll be plugged into a support system that can get you the help you need.

Time for a Change

To prevent eating disorders, a potentially fatal disease, we must change the way we judge ourselves and others and the demands and unrealistic goals we set. We are rewarded for looking good far more frequently than being good or being smart. This is particularly true for young women. People are judged-literally-at face value. To turn the tide, try to shoot for these goals:

Use Your Time Wisely.

Time well spent is time used for analyzing important issues and charting your future. Time spent counting fat grams and searching out body flaws is a different matter. College is a critically important time to take care of your body so that it can take care of you and help you meet the challenges of school. This means developing healthy eating habits and a healthy body image. Liberate yourself from the negative, body-bashing, dieting experiences that bond some women. Get a handle on who you are inside as opposed to who you are on the outside, and nurture/pamper yourself from the inside out.

Be Critical of Messages and Images in the Media.

Look beyond magazines and television to find normal bodies. Don't equate healthy with being bone-thin. Instead, focus on eating well, being active, and having fun.

Find Some Normal-looking Role Models.

It's a challenge to find role models who like their bodies, eat normally, and exercise moderately, but they do exist. Learn to accept diversity of shape and size, and evaluate success by accomplishments rather than a number on the scale.

FOR MORE INFORMATION . . .

Books

Anderson, A., L. Cohen and T. Holbrook., 2000. *Making Weight: Men's Conflicts with Food, Weight, Shape and Appearance.* California: Gurze Publications.

Berg, F. 2001. Children and Teens Afraid to Eat: Helping Youth in Today's Weight Obsessed World, *Healthy Weight Journal.*

Brumberg, J. 1997. *The Body Project: An Intimate History of American Girls.* New York: Random House.

Koenig, K. *The Rules of Normal Eating: A Commonsense Approach for Dieters, Overeaters, Undereaters, Emotional Eaters, and Everyone in Between.* California: Gurze Publications.

Tribole, E., and E. Resch. 2003. *Intuitive Eating; A Recovery Book for the Chronic Dieter.* New York: St. Martin's Press.

Organizations and Resources

Somethingfishy: Online resource
www.something-fishy.com

Eating Disorder Referral and Information Center
www.edreferral.com

Resources, information and support for eating disorders
www.bulimia.com

Find a Registered Dietitian
www.eatright.org.

Renfrew Treatment Center
www.renfrew.org

International Association of Eating Disorders Professionals
www.iaedp.com

PART III
Challenges to Eating Well in College

CHAPTER

8

Vegging Out

Vegetarianism is hot. Once considered a left-wing, fanatical life-style, vegetarian diets have gone mainstream and continue to receive hearty endorsements from various health organizations.

Vegetarian diets have been around since the beginning of time, but over the past few years they have attracted an increasing number of fans. The growing popularity of vegetarian diets is good news since it makes non-meat alternatives more available. Take a look at a typical restaurant menu. Even chain restaurants, such as T.G.I.Fridays, Ruby Tuesday, and Subway are onto the trend and include veggie meals on their menus.

Why Become a Vegetarian?

People become vegetarians for many reasons. The thought of eating "anything that once breathed" is a motivating factor for some, while religious beliefs are for others. Some people choose to be vegetarian because a plant-based diet is considered better for the environment. Raising animals for food does use up many natural resources such as water and arable land. Another compelling reason to eat a vegetarian diet is that it means you eat "lower on the food chain." If the grain used to fatten up animals that are then slaughtered for human consumption were used to feed hungry people instead, a lot could be done to alleviate world hunger.

The recent interest in vegetarianism, however, seems to be more associated with a personal interest in health. News reports about the benefits of eating more fruits, vegetables, and grains are on the increase while, in contrast, stories about meat are less encouraging. The concerns surrounding the safety of meat and the health problems associated with eating too much fat (meat can be a significant source of fat) make vegetarianism a desirable choice for many.

Eating a vegetarian diet can be a healthy move, but it doesn't guarantee that your diet will be a nutritional winner. Unless properly planned, the diet may be unbalanced and lacking in certain critical nutrients.

Occasionally, adopting a vegetarian diet is used as a way to mask an underlying eating disorder. Being a vegetarian becomes a legitimate reason, one that won't be challenged, to exclude whole categories of food. Generally, the eating disordered vegetarian diet is very rigid and excludes not only animal products, but other high-calorie or high-fat foods as well. The truly committed vegetarian is willing to include a wide variety of animal-free foods, even those that may be higher in fat and calories.

The Food Guide Pyramid—the pictorial view of how health experts suggest Americans eat—backs up the argument for choosing a more plant-based diet. (see Chart 1–14). Add together the recommended number of servings of foods you should eat from grains, fruits and vegetables and it's pretty clear: plants rule and should make up the lion's share of what everyone, not only the vegetarian, eats.

Types of Vegetarian Diets

There are many types of vegetarians. Ask a few friends who claim to be vegetarians what they eat, and you're likely to get different answers from each.

The actual definition of a vegetarian is "someone who avoids all meat, including fish and poultry." But most individuals who consider themselves "plant people," or vegetarians, eat animal-based foods at least to some extent (see Chart 8–1).

CHART 8–1

Different Types of Vegetarians

LACTO-OVO VEGETARIAN: excludes meat, poultry, and fish but eats dairy products and eggs.

LACTO VEGETARIAN: excludes meat, poultry, fish, and eggs but includes dairy products.

STRICT VEGETARIAN OR VEGAN: excludes all animal products, including meat, poultry, fish, eggs, and dairy products. Some vegans also exclude honey.

Eating the Vegetarian Way

Whether you eat a vegetarian diet or not, it helps to be conscientious about your food choices. The key concern with a vegetarian diet is that, once you eliminate a food group, you eliminate certain vitamins, minerals, and other nutrients common to that group. The more foods you eliminate, the more likely you'll lack certain vitamins and minerals. Armed with accurate nutrition information, however, the potential problems with a vegetarian diet can be avoided.

Protein

Since animal foods are excellent sources of protein, if you remove some or all animal foods from your diet do you run into a protein problem? It's rare that a vegetarian doesn't get enough protein (see

Chart 8–2). All animal foods, including dairy products and eggs, contain high-quality protein. If you are a lacto-ovo, or lacto vegetarian, you don't need to be concerned about your protein intake.

Even for vegans, people who eat nothing but plant-based foods, protein is seldom a problem. Plants are rich in protein. Beans and legumes, such as kidney beans, chickpeas, navy beans, lentils, soybeans, nuts, and seeds, are just a few examples of non-meat protein. Some of these foods such as peanut butter, peas, and kidney beans may already be a part of your diet. Others such as navy beans, lentils or tofu, may be less familiar (see Chart 8–3).

CHART 8–2

How's Your Protein Intake

	Age	
	15–18	19–24
Female	44 gms/day	46 gms/day
Male	59 gms/day	58 gms/day

- Record all of the food and amounts that you eat in a typical day.
- Consult Chart 8–3 for the amount of protein found in foods that are considered good protein sources.
- Tally up your protein intake in a day and compare it to the amount you need.

Animal and non-animal proteins vary in their quality. All animal proteins, including dairy, eggs, and cheese provide the amino acid pattern that is perfect for our bodies to use. The proteins in plant based foods such as beans, peas, and wheat, have varying amounts of amino acids. Nutrition experts used to think that you had to combine different plant-based foods such as nuts and wheat or rice and beans, to get the kind of complete protein the body needed. The protein pattern formed by eating these foods together was termed "complementary protein." However, we now know that when the diet is adequate in calories, includes rich sources of plant protein, and contains a variety of foods, complementing proteins is not necessary.

CHART 8–3

Sources of Protein

FOOD	SERVING	PROTEIN (gm)/CALORIES
Animal Protein		
Boneless, skinless chicken breast	½ breast	26 / 140
Canned tuna	3 oz. (small can)	22 / 100
Skim milk	8 oz.	8 / 80
Vanilla yogurt	6 oz. (small carton)	9 / 180
Egg	1	6 / 75
Hard cheese	1 oz. (1" cube)	7 / 110
Cottage cheese	½ cup	14 / 80
Sirloin steak	6 oz.	51 / 308
Hamburger	4 oz. patty	33 / 292
Flounder	4 oz.	23 / 113
Shrimp	6 large	8.5 / 45
Cheese pizza	1 slice	14 / 200
Non-meat Protein		
Peanut butter	2 Tbsp.	8 / 188
Chickpeas	½ cup	6 / 140
Black beans	½ cup	7 / 162
Pasta	1½ cup	10 / 300
Brown rice	1 cup	5 / 220
White rice	1 cup	5 / 240
Baked potato	1	4 / 220
Hummus	3 Tbsp.	3 / 105
Tofu	½ cup	20 / 183
Garden/veggie burger	1	8 / 140
Boca burger	1	12 / 84
Bagel	1 large	10 / 270
Lentil soup	1 mug	9 / 140
Minestrone soup	1 mug	5 / 120
Black bean soup	1 mug	8 / 170
Enriched soy beverage	8 oz.	9 / 130
Rice beverage	8 oz.	1 / 90
Tofu "hotdog"	1	9 / 45
Fast food bean burrito	1	13 / 370
Power Bar	1	10 / 230
Balance Bar	1	14 / 180
Clif Bar	1	12 / 250

CHART 8–4

Sources of Calcium

FOOD	SERVING	CALCIUM (mg)
Skim milk	8 oz.	300
Yogurt	8 oz. carton	400
Hard cheese	1" cube	200
Cottage cheese	½ cup	75
Cheese pizza	1 slice	150
Broccoli	½ cup cooked	45
Kale, collard greens	½ cup cooked	90
Calcium-fortified orange juice	8 oz.	300
Calcium-fortified soy milk	8 oz.	240
Calcium-fortified string cheese	1 piece	250
Calcium-fortified cereal	1 cup	250
Ice cream, soft serve	6 oz./small	90–120
Ice cream, hard	1 scoop	80–90
Frozen yogurt, soft serve	6 oz./small	100–130

Minerals

Calcium, **iron**, and **zinc** are nutrients found primarily in animal foods. **Calcium** is critical for developing and maintaining strong bones and teeth and regulating heartbeat and muscle contractions. Even though most college-age students have finished growing and building bones, calcium intake remains important throughout your life. Peak bone mass doesn't occur until you're in your 30s, and bodies naturally lose calcium throughout your lifetime.

Iron is involved in carrying oxygen in the body, and **zinc** is involved in many crucial bodily processes. Without enough iron, you could develop iron-deficiency anemia, a condition that will make you feel tired and run down. Without enough zinc, you may be more susceptible to infections.

The lacto-ovo and lacto vegetarian can easily meet their **calcium** needs by getting two to three servings of **dairy foods** a day. If dairy products are omitted, vegetables such as **broccoli, bok choy (Chinese cabbage) kale, collards,** and **mustard greens** are good sources of calcium. You're not likely to find these foods regularly on campus, so you may need to include calcium-fortified foods such as **calcium-fortified orange juice**, some **ready-to-eat cereals**, **tofu**, and **soy milk** to meet your calcium needs (see Chart 8–4).

For non-vegetarians, meat usually provides **iron** and **zinc**. Vegetarians need to look for other ways to include these essential minerals in their diets. One of the easiest and most reliable ways to get enough iron and zinc is to have a **fortified breakfast cereal. Dried beans, dried fruit, seeds,** and **prune juice** are good plant sources of iron and zinc. Iron from plant sources will be absorbed better if you eat them with foods rich in vitamin C such as citrus fruits, tomatoes, broccoli, and melons (see Chart 8–5). If you're preparing your own food, you can boost your iron intake by cooking with a cast iron pan. Some iron leaches out into the food and can be absorbed and used by your body.

Vitamins

If your diet excludes all meat and dairy foods, **vitamin B12** and **vitamin D** will likely be in short supply. **Vitamin B12** is necessary to

---

CHART 8–5

Sources of Iron and Zinc

FOOD	SERVING	IRON (mg)	ZINC (mg)
Hamburger	4 oz. patty	2.5	6.0
Boneless chicken breast	4 oz.	0.89	0.86
Canned tuna	3 oz. can	1.3	0.65
Cereal			
Total	1 cup	18.0	0.67
Cheerios	1¼ cup	4.45	0.79
Cornflakes	1 cup	1.8	0.9
Bran flakes	¾ cup	18.0	3.75
Cream of Wheat	1 cup, cooked	9.0	0.31
Instant oatmeal	1 packet	8.35	0.88
Garbanzo beans	½ cup	1.65	1.25
Lentil soup	1 bowl	4.2	
Minestrone soup	1 bowl	1.4	

keep your blood healthy. Without adequate amounts of this vitamin, you could suffer irreversible nerve damage. **Vitamin B**12 is found in **all animal products**, so if you're a lacto-ovo vegetarian you shouldn't have a problem taking in enough. Vegans will need to look for foods fortified with **vitamin B**12 such as **soy milk**, **breakfast cereals**, and **fortified vegetarian nutritional yeasts.**

Vitamin D is necessary for calcium and other nutrients to be absorbed. Without it, you increase the risk of bone disease later in life; however, **vitamin D** doesn't occur naturally in food. People have relied on the sun to convert the body's own inactive form of **vitamin D** into a usable form. But, as people spend more time indoors, their exposure to the sun has become more limited. To ensure that Americans get enough **vitamin D** in their diet, all fluid cow's milk is routinely fortified with it. If you're not a milk drinker, you can also get **vitamin D** from **fortified soy milk** and **certain breakfast cereals**.

Supplements

Taking a vitamin and mineral supplement is no cure for a poorly planned diet. However, if you review the food sources for those nutrients that are potentially limited for vegetarians, or if you know those foods aren't available to you, you may want to consider using a multivitamin supplement to cover yourself (see the discussion about vitamins in Chapter 1).

Fat

Following a vegetarian diet is not necessarily a healthy, low-fat diet unless you make good food choices. Many vegetarians tend to rely on high-fat cheese, high-fat processed soy products, and go heavy on nuts and seeds. While these are excellent vegetarian foods, follow the servings recommended in the food pyramid (see Chart 1–13) so your diet doesn't become laden with too much fat.

CHART 8–6

Typical Vegetarian Meals on Campus

Lacto-ovo vegetarian

Breakfast
  Total cereal, milk, banana, toast with margarine
Lunch
  Veggie burger on a bun
  Vegetable soup
Snack
  Vanilla yogurt
Dinner
  Cheese-filled pasta with cooked vegetables
  Skim milk and Oreos
Snack
  2 slices of toast with spread, hot herbal tea

Total: 2050 calories, 98 gm protein, 52 gm fat, 311 gm carbohydrate. Adequate in all major nutrients.

Breakfast
  2 packages of instant oatmeal with raisins
  Calcium-fortified orange juice
Lunch
  Pizza bagel, water
Snack
  Cheerios cereal and milk
Dinner
  Stir-fry veggies and tofu over rice
  Apple
  Frozen yogurt

Total: 1500 calories, 64 gm protein, 21 gm fat, 279 gm carbohydrate. Adequate in all major nutrients except Vitamin E and a bit too low in fat. To improve: Add a small amount of margarine or salad oil.

Breakfast
  (Missed)
Lunch
  Lentil soup, bagel, banana
Snack
  2 pieces string cheese and an apple
Dinner
  Large salad with lettuce, carrots, cucumbers, green peppers, hard-boiled eggs, cottage cheese
  Fruit juice
  Baked potato with plain yogurt
  Dinner roll
Snack
  2 slices plain pizza

Total: 1700 calories, 83 gm protein, 38 gm fat, 258 gm carbohydrate. Adequate in all major nutrients except vitamin E. To improve: Add small amount of salad oil or margarine.

Vegan

Breakfast
  Total cereal, fortified soy milk
Lunch
  Pita bread stuffed with hummus and vegetables
  Fruit
  Black bean soup
Snack
  Trail mix and fruit smoothie
Dinner
  Stir-fried veggies with tofu over rice
  Salad
  Sorbet
Snack
  Toast with honey and fortified soy milk

Total: 2200 calories, 62 gm protein, 32 gm fat, 439 gm carbohydrate. Adequate in all major nutrients.

Breakfast
  Bagel with jam, calcium-fortified orange juice
Lunch
  Peanut butter sandwich, fruit, juice
Snack
  Lentil soup and juice
Dinner
  Pasta with veggies and tomato sauce
  Roll
  Calcium-fortified orange juice

Total: 1900 Calories, 55 gm protein, 25 gm fat, 377 gm carbohydrate. Adequate in most major nutrients. Slightly low in zinc, and some B vitamins. To improve: add a serving of fortified breakfast cereal.

Breakfast
  Hot cereal, fortified soy beverage, fruit
Lunch
  Bean burrito, salad, juice
Snack
  English muffin with peanut butter
Dinner
  Veggie burger, roll, cooked vegetables, salad with tofu chunks
  Sorbet
Snack
  Bagel and fruit smoothie

Total: 2100 calories, 67 gm protein, 36 gm fat, 382 gm carbohydrate. Inadequate in calcium. To improve: add calcium-fortified orange juice.

Making Your Food Choices

Thanks to the growing popularity of vegetarian diets, you can now find a variety of vegetarian foods on most campuses (see Chart 8–6). Typical cafeteria entrees often include:

- Pasta
- Meatless chili and soups
- Stir-fry dishes
- Veggie burgers
- Eggs
- Peanut butter and jelly
- Vegetarian burritos and wraps
- Pizza

As with all diets, what you choose to eat and how much are key to a balanced diet. You may not be familiar with some of these foods on the vegetarian pyramid, but with an open and adventurous attitude, you can discover the limitless possibilities plant foods offer.

Don't assume that just because you're eating a vegetarian diet it's automatically a healthier diet. It will require a little extra effort in planning. But eating a vegetarian diet can be more than nutritionally adequate, incredibly healthy, and, above all, delicious. You may also make a small contribution to a healthier world.

FOR MORE INFORMATION . . .

Books

Dorfman, L. 2000. *The Vegetarian Sports Nutrition Guide : Peak Performance for Everyone from Beginners to Gold Medalists.* New York: John Wiley.

Havala, S. 2001. *Being Vegetarian for Dummies.* New York: John Wiley

Melina, V. and Davis, B. 2003. *The New Becoming Vegetarian: The Essential Guide to a Healthy Vegetarian Diet.* Summertown, TN: Healthy Living Publication

Organizations and Resources

The Vegetarian Resource Group
www.vrg.org

Vegetarian Times
www.vegetariantimes.com

CHAPTER

Eating To Compete

Whether you're a competitive athlete, a weekend sports warrior, or someone who simply works out to stay in shape, how you fuel your body can make a big difference in how it performs. For competitive athletes, that difference can make or break their success on the field or in the gym.

Every sport places different demands on the body. While there is no single magic bullet to replace natural talent and good old-fashioned training, eating right can help you perform at your best, reduce your risk of injury, and delay the onset of fatigue.

The basic diet for an athlete is essentially the same as the basic diet for a non-athlete. The difference is that athletes need more of everything . . . **more calories, more protein, more vitamins, more minerals, more fluids**. Knowing what, when, and how much to eat before, during, and after training and competing can give you the winning edge.

Calories

Your calorie needs during training and exercise are determined by:

- Your height;
- Your weight;
- Your gender;
- Your age;
- Your body composition;
- Your level of fitness;
- How hard, how long, and how often you exercise.

Obviously, a 6'5" 240-pound basketball player needs more food than a 5'1" 103-pound gymnast, and a long distance runner has different needs than a sprinter. To get an idea of how many calories you might burn while participating in different activities, see Chart 9–1.

Protein, fat, and carbohydrate all provide your body with **calories**— the fuel your body uses to perform. There are significant differences in how your body burns protein, fat, and carbohydrate. Some are more immediate fuel sources than others, so what you choose to eat will affect how you feel when exercising.

Carbohydrates

The Fuel of Choice

When you exercise, your body prefers carbohydrates as its primary source of fuel or energy. Carbohydrates are easily digested, absorbed, and converted to blood sugar, which is then immediately available for your active muscles to use.

Types of Carbohydrate Foods to Include

Simple carbohydrates such as **candy**, **soda**, **fruit**, and **fruit juice**, are digested and absorbed more quickly than the **complex carbohydrates** such as **cereals** and **whole grain breads**. But you can't survive

---

CHART 9–1

Calories Expended in Sports

SPORT	CALORIES BURNED PER MINUTE FOR ACTIVITY*			
	110 lb.	130 lb.	150 lb.	170 lb.
Baseball				
Player	3.4	4.1	4.7	5.3
Pitcher	4.3	5.1	5.9	6.7
Basketball	7.2	8.5	9.9	11.2
Biking				
5 mph	2.1	2.5	2.9	3.3
10 mph	4.6	5.5	6.4	7.2
15 mph	8.0	9.5	10.9	12.4
Fencing	7.3	8.7	10.0	11.4
Football	6.1	7.2	8.3	9.4
Golf	4.0	4.7	5.4	6.2
Gymnastics, dancing	6.7	7.9	9.1	10.3
Hockey				
Field	6.7	7.9	9.1	10.3
Ice	7.3	8.7	10.0	11.4
Rollerblading	4.6	5.5	6.4	7.2
Running				
5 mph	6.6	7.9	9.1	10.3
7 mph	9.3	11.0	12.8	14.5
9 mph	11.9	14.0	16.2	18.4
12 mph	16.0	18.9	21.9	24.8
Skiing, cross-country				
2.5 mph	5.5	6.5	7.5	8.5
5 mph	8.4	10.0	11.5	13.1
Skiing, downhill	7.2	8.5	9.9	11.2
Soccer	6.6	7.8	9.0	10.2
Swimming				
Backstroke				
30 yds/min	3.9	4.6	5.3	6.0
40 yds/min	6.1	7.2	8.3	9.4
Breastroke				
30 yds/min	5.2	6.2	7.1	8.1
40 yds/min	7.0	8.3	9.6	10.9
Crawl				
25 yds/min	4.4	5.2	6.0	6.8
50 yds/min	7.7	9.2	10.6	12.0
Table tennis	3.8	4.5	5.2	5.9
Tennis, singles	7.1	8.4	9.8	11.1
Volleyball	7.1	8.4	9.8	11.1
Walking				
3 mph	3.0	3.5	4.1	4.6
4 mph	4.6	5.5	6.4	7.2
5 mph	6.0	7.1	8.2	9.2
Weightlifting	5.7	6.8	7.8	8.9
Wrestling	9.3	11.1	12.8	14.8

*The values expressed here are averages and vary depending on conditions such as terrain, weather, wind resistance, etc. It is assumed that all sports are being done competitively

Adapted from: Coleman, E. and S. N. Steen. *The Ultimate Sports Nutrition Handbook*. 1996. Palo Alto, Ca. Bull Publishing.

on sweet-tasting sugars because they contain few nutrients, yet they pack plenty of calories. To be sure you get the nutrients you need to grow muscle tissue, strengthen bones, increase oxygen capacity, and have optimum energy, you should eat simple sugars in addition to, not in place of, the more nutrient-rich complex carbohydrates.

Carbohydrate Loading

Not all of the carbohydrates you eat are used immediately for energy; some are stored in your muscles and your liver. This storage form of carbohydrates is called **glycogen**. Endurance athletes (see Chart 9–2) rely on glycogen to fuel their prolonged energy needs. Although we store far more calories as fat, muscles prefer to use carbohydrates as fuel.

The muscles can only store a limited amount of glycogen, but, for short periods of time, they can become super-saturated with glycogen.

CHART 9–2

Endurance or Non-Endurance?

Endurance sports are those that last 60-90 minutes or longer:
- Cross-country running
- Long distance biking
- Field hockey
- Marathons
- Triathlons
- Cross-country skiing
- Long distance swimming
- Soccer
- Biathlons

Non-endurance sports generally require short bursts of energy. They may go on for an hour or more, and they may be of high or low intensity:
- Baseball
- Golf
- Sprinting (swimming, running)
- Volleyball
- Gymnastics
- Softball
- Speed skating
- Tennis
- Weightlifting

Some sports straddle both, depending on duration and amount of playing time:
- Football
- Ice hockey
- Swimming
- Basketball
- Tennis
- Soccer

Athletes can effectively increase their stores of glycogen by following a training and diet regime known as **carbohydrate loading** or **carbo loading**. By maximizing glycogen stores, you can increase the amount of glucose available to your muscles for fuel which can delay the onset of fatigue. Carbo loading works best for bodies that are trained. Weekend athletes find little benefit from carbo loading (see Chart 9–3).

The term "hitting the wall" is infamous and dreaded among athletes. Scientifically it means that you've exhausted just about all of the glycogen stored in your muscles and you feel completely "out of gas." When you've used up all of the liver glycogen, your brain feels the effect, rather than your body. You may feel lightheaded and even disoriented. Unlike muscles that can draw on fat for energy once glycogen is used, the brain likes only glucose. To avoid problems, athletes should learn

---

CHART 9–3

Carbohydrate-Loading Formula

To increase your glycogen stores, you must **continuously** eat right and train hard, not just prior to an event. Carbohydrate loading will only benefit the trained athlete. It won't make athletes faster, it just allows glucose storage for use over a longer period of time. To increase stores:

7-10 DAYS BEFORE EVENT
- Gradually reduce training or taper off. This will allow your muscles to rest and "load" with carbohydrates.
- Since you'll be training less, you don't need to eat more food, just the same amount you've been eating all along.

3 DAYS BEFORE EVENT
- Increase your intake of fiber-rich, complex carbohydrate foods: whole grain cereal; beans; starchy vegetables like potatoes, corn, peas; whole wheat breads, fruit, and veggies. If you rely mainly on pasta, which is not fiber-rich, you may become constipated because you've decreased your training.
- Be sure to take in enough fluids and protein to prevent constipation.

DAY OF EVENT
- Eat food you know will digest and settle well.
- Avoid fruit, since it may give you diarrhea.
- Pay attention to your fluid needs.
- Don't try anything new!

to eat something just before their event so the brain receives the glucose it needs to perform optimally (see Chart 9–8).

Fat

Fat Burning During Exercise

Your body burns fat during exercise, too. The mix of glycogen and fat used to meet energy needs depends on the type of exercise you do and how long you do it. For example, fat is the primary source of fuel in low-intensity exercising such as walking. In endurance sports, like biking or long distance running, glycogen is the primary source of energy and then fat. But in sports where energy bursts are short, intense, and repeated often such as tennis, soccer, or hockey, carbohydrates (glycogen) is the main source of fuel and fat isn't used much for energy.

Since excess protein, fat, and carbs are stored as body fat, you rarely need to eat extra fat to increase fat stores, which, in turn, can be used for energy. For good health, athletes and non-athletes alike should strive to eat about 20-30 percent of their total calories in the form of fat (see Chart 9-4).

CHART 9–4

Sensible Eating Plan for the College Athlete

BREAKFAST
Bagel/cream cheese
Fruit juice

LUNCH
Turkey sub
Fruit
Skim milk
Small bag of chips

SNACK
Fruit Smoothie
Granola bar

DINNER
Roasted chicken breast
Baked potato with margarine
Veggies
Water
Roll and margarine

SNACK
Cereal and milk

2600 calories, 20% protein, 20% fat, 60% carbohydrate.

Body Fat

Highly trained athletes usually have very little body fat because intense training burns excess calories, leaving little to be stored as fat (see Chart 9–5). Regardless of the focus on "fat free," some dietary fat and body fat are necessary for good health and optimal performance. For example, body fat is needed to regulate body temperature. If you don't have enough fat on your body, you're more likely to become dehydrated and fatigued.

CHART 9–5

Ranges of Percent of Body Fat in Competitive Athletes

SPORT	MEN	WOMEN
Biking	5–11%	8–15%
Football	6–18%	*
Golf	10–16%	12–20%
Gymnastics	5–12%	8–16%
Ice and field hockey	8–16%	12–18%
Rowing	6–14%	8–16%
Running	5–12%	8–15%
Skiing	7–15%	10–18%
Soccer	6–14%	10–18%
Swimming	6–12%	10–18%
Tennis	6–14%	10–20%
Volleyball	7–15%	10–18%
Weightlifting	5–12%	10–18%
Wrestling	5–16%	*

*Data not available

Adapted from: Wilmore, J. and D. Costill. 1994. *Physiology of Sport and Exercise* Champaign, IL: Human Kinetics.

For the female athlete, a low percentage of body fat, too little fat in the diet, and intense training can cause menstruation to stop. The non-menstruating female athlete is at a much higher risk for fractures and thinning or weakening of bones. To prevent long-term, irreversible losses in bone density, female athletes at risk should eat a higher-fat diet, and, perhaps, lighten their training schedules.

Protein

Protein Requirements

Protein is the building block of muscles. Athletes need more protein in their diets than non-athletes (see Chart 9–6). Our diets provide plenty of protein, so it's easy to get this additional amount by eating "regular" food, rather than special supplements or powders. Even those with the highest protein needs should be able to meet them with food (see Chart 8–3).

CHART 9–6

Protein Requirements

	GRAMS OF PROTEIN/LB. OF BODY WEIGHT
Current RDA sedentary adult	0.4
Competitive athlete, still growing	0.8–0.9
Recreational athlete	0.5–0.75
Competitive athlete, no longer growing	0.6–0.9
Weight lifter	0.7–0.9

Adapted with permission from Nancy Clark, 1997, *Nancy Clark's Sports Nutrition Guidebook*, 2nd ed. Champaign, IL: Human Kinetics, 131.

Too much or just right?

Many athletes are tempted to use amino acid and protein supplements. Keep in mind, however, that there's no evidence that exceeding the recommended ranges of protein intake will increase muscle size or performance. Eating excess protein doesn't build big bulging muscles and can actually be harmful because it places too much strain on your kidneys. The right amount of protein and training is what boosts bulk. And protein is readily available in our food supply.

When you eat more protein than your body needs for muscle building and other uses, some will be burned for energy. However, the rest ends up like any other extra calories you consume. You store extra protein as body fat.

Vitamins and Minerals

Vitamins and minerals help your body use the food you eat. They don't contain calories. Since athletes eat more food because they have higher energy needs, and they burn more calories through their extra exercise/activity, it's logical to think that athletes need more vitamins and minerals, too. Just by eating more food, athletes can get the extra vitamins and minerals they need.

An exception to this rule is in the case of athletes participating in endurance sports. Hard-core training can increase the amount of iron your body loses. If you don't eat an iron-rich diet (see Chart 8–5), if you're a menstruating woman who loses iron each month, or you're an endurance athlete, you may be at greater risk for iron-deficiency anemia. The most common symptom of anemia is fatigue. Left untreated, anemia can be debilitating. Endurance athletes should have their iron levels checked periodically.

Female athletes should also evaluate their calcium intake, which is often limited in women's diets. Lack of calcium may not produce immediate symptoms, but it can eventually contribute to bone loss (see Chart 8-4).

Fluids and Electrolytes

Functions of Fluids

Fluids are the most important part of an athlete's diet. Fluids help move glucose and other nutrients through the body to exercising muscles, and they remove wastes from the body through the production of urine.

Fluids are responsible for the body's ability to regulate its internal temperature. During exercise, the body heats up and sweats. Sweat is made up of water with a small amount of sodium, potassium, and other electrolytes mixed in. As sweat evaporates, the body cools down. Replacing fluids lost through sweat is essential to regulate body temperature and to keep electrolytes in balance. If you don't replace fluids, your performance will be impaired and you can face serious dehydration problems such as heat cramps, heat exhaustion, or heat stroke (see Chart 9–7).

You lose small amounts of electrolytes when you sweat, most of which is sodium. This sodium needs to be replaced, but because it's abundant in the average diet, running low on sodium is rare. Eating salty foods or sprinkling some salt on your food will replace sodium. **Salt tablets are unnecessary**.

CHART 9- 7

Are You Drinking Enough?

Thirst is never a reliable indicator of an athlete's need for fluid. To be well hydrated, you must **drink before, during, and after exercising . . . and then drink some more**. If you're drinking enough, you should:

- Urinate often
- Your urine should be a clear, pale yellow.

In its mildest form, dehydration makes you feel tired and uncomfortable and impairs your performance. In severe cases, it can kill you. Watch for these signs of dehydration:

- Dry mouth, chills, heat cramps, fatigue, headache;
- GI problems, such as nausea, dizziness, confusion, increased weakness; and
- Extreme thirst with no urine output, hallucinations, swollen tongue, high body temperature.

Fluid guidelines
- Drink extra fluids the day before an event, and shoot for at least eight 8 oz. glasses.
- Drink 16–20 oz. of fluids 2–2½ hours before the event.
- Drink another 8–16 oz. right before the event starts.
- During the event, drink as much as you can. Try to drink 8 oz. every 15 minutes.
- After the event, drink as much as you need to replace the fluids lost.

Getting Enough

It makes sense to drink when you're thirsty, but you can't rely on thirst alone to tell you to drink. In fact, exercise can delay your thirst signal to the brain so that by the time you feel thirsty, you may lose as much as one percent of your body weight. Dehydration sets in, and your performance is affected when you don't drink enough. To avoid problems, it makes sense to establish a pattern for consuming fluids.

You can monitor fluid adequacy by the color of your urine and how often you urinate. Urine should be a clear yellow, not dark. You should urinate frequently throughout the day. If it's dark and/or you're not urinating often, double up on fluids.

Choosing What to Drink

Water, fruit juice, vegetable juice, and sports drinks all provide fluid in your diet. If you're working out or participating in an event that lasts less than 60 minutes, water is the fluid of choice, although sports drinks are fine. If you're in events lasting longer than 60 minutes, sports drinks are a good choice because they contain carbohydrates to help nourish your working muscles and delay fatigue.

Fruit juices and sodas are concentrated sources of sugar. Drinking too much of them while exercising can cause cramping, diarrhea, and nausea. Therefore, use sugar-rich drinks carefully before endurance events. If you prefer to drink fruit juice or soda, try diluting them with varying amounts of water until you find a formula that works for you.

The Other Fluids . . . Caffeine and Alcohol

Caffeine-containing beverages such as coffee and colas, and alcoholic beverages are generally not great choices to replace fluid losses. Caffeine and alcohol act like a diuretic and increase fluid loss. Beer and alcohol can cause you to urinate more, making fluid losses even greater. Alcohol and beer also interfere with your balance and coordination, which can have an obvious impact on your performance.

There are conflicting studies on caffeine's effect on athletic performance. At one time, caffeine was reported to mobilize fat and thus

increase fat burning by the muscles. This has never been proven scientifically. Caffeine seems to make some people feel more alert and
focused. It can make others jittery, cause headaches, and stomach
upsets (more about caffeine in Chapter 11). And, as mentioned ear-
lier, it can act as a diuretic and promote dehydration. Know your limit
and how caffeinated drinks make you feel. At the very least, be sure to
drink plenty of non-caffeinated fluids to prevent dehydration.

Meal Planning for Events

For competitive athletes, knowing what to eat is only one part of the
plan. Knowing when to eat before, during, and after an event is crucial
too.

What to eat before an event varies from sport to sport and athlete to
athlete. There are no hard and fast rules about what works, but some
general guidelines do apply. Whatever you do, don't experiment on the
day of the event. Instead, try out different foods and vary when you eat
them during training to see what feels best (see Chart 9–8).

Before

The **pre-competition meal** should provide you with enough energy
to perform well and delay premature fatigue. It shouldn't, however,
make you feel too full or cause digestive problems. Keep in mind, too,
that being anxious or nervous prior to competition will affect how you
digest foods.

Timing of meals is essential. **Large meals take three to four hours
to digest; smaller ones take about two to three hours**. Plan your
meals accordingly. Most athletes feel comfortable eating two to four
hours before competing. If the event is early in the morning, a smaller
meal usually works well. If you're competing/performing later in the
day, you may be able to eat a hearty breakfast and then a light lunch or
snack.

Generally, carbohydrate-rich foods are the best choice for a pre-
event meal because they are digested and absorbed the quickest and

CHART 9–8

"Balanced Bars"

Many college students . . . athletes and non-athletes wonder about the various "sports bars" and "energy bars". While a good homemade snack will fit the bill, the bars tend to be more nutritious than a candy bar—and portable. Here's how some popular bars stack up:

PRODUCT	CALORIES*	PROTEIN	CHO	FAT	COMMENTS
Balance	200	14	22	6	Pre and post workout
Balance Gold	210	15	23	7	Pre and post workout
Balance Outdoor	200	15	21	6	Pre and post workout
Clif	230	10	41	4	Pre workout/endurance
Luna	180	10	25	4	Pre and post workout
Met-Rx Food Bar	320	27	48	2.5	Post workout/meal
Odwalla	240	7	48	4	Pre workout/short duration
PowerBar Harvest	240	7	45	4	Pre workout/short duration
PowerBar Performance	230	10	45	3	Pre workout/short duration
FOR COMPARISON					
Nutrigrain bar	140	2	27	3	Pre workout/short duration
Granola bar	120	2	21	3	Pre workout/short duration
Snicker's bar	280	4	35	14	

*adapted from Raising the Bar, *Nutrition Action Healthletter*, December, 2000 and Fuel for Young Athletes, *Human Kinetics* 2004.

easiest (see Chart 9–9). Your body can't digest and absorb a high protein meal as quickly and may cause indigestion or nausea later on. High-fat foods tend to stay in the stomach the longest and may make you feel uncomfortable. The protein and fat rich steak and egg breakfast is best eaten on a day off.

If you can't eat a meal, a small snack one to two hours before the event may combat hunger, give you energy, and maintain your blood sugar level. Select a carbohydrate-rich food or consider a blenderized beverage, since liquids are absorbed more quickly than solid foods.

Finally, pre-competition meals often are as important for your mind as they are for your body. If you think something helps you perform better, break the rules and eat it.

CHART 9–9

Carbohydrate-Rich Foods

FOOD	SERVING	CARBOHYDRATE (gm)
Bagel	1 bakery size	50
Bran/blueberry muffin	1 medium	20
Baked potato	1 medium	50
Rice	1 cup	36
Pasta	2 cups	88
Oatmeal, instant	1 packet	19
Flaked cereal	3 handfuls	40
Apple, orange, banana	1	15–25
Raisins	1 small box	30
Dried apricots	7–10	20–25
100% fruit juice	8 oz.	20–30
Sports drinks	8 oz.	20–30
Power Bar	1	45
Balance Bar	1	22
Granola Bar	1	20-30
Cliff Bar	1	40

During

Getting enough fluid is the most important concern during an event. If you're participating in an event that lasts longer than 60 minutes, you may find sports drinks, sports "goo," or other easily digested carbohydrate foods useful. At the very least, drink fluids every 15 minutes.

If your event is 60 minutes or longer, or if you're competing in a series of events spread over many hours such as a swim meet, regatta, or soccer tournament, consider eating small, carbohydrate-rich snacks throughout the event. Your body needs food to help maintain blood sugar levels. Experiment to see how much your body can handle comfortably while you're exercising.

After

With so much focus on what to eat and drink before and during an event or training, we often forget the importance of the post-event meal. Refeeding tired muscles has a profound effect on how you feel. If you're often exhausted from training, pay greater attention to your post-event diet.

What you eat within the first few minutes after a workout or competition is known as **recovery eating.** First and foremost, drink plenty of fluids. But eating is important, too. 15 to 30 minutes after exercising, the muscles are like sponges waiting to refill those glycogen stores that have just been used. Refuel your muscles with what they like best: a combination of a carbohydrate rich food with some protein. In real food terms, this might be a peanut butter sandwich and a glass of chocolate milk, a banana and string cheese or a carton of yogurt and some crackers.

Many athletes just can't eat or don't want to eat right after exercise. A good compromise is to drink a commercial recovery drink with added protein. Unfortunately, some athletes who are interested in losing weight don't want to eat right after exercising, because they are not interested in replacing the calories they just "burned". In fact, recovery eating will help keep them from bingeing later on in the day. Remember, this is just a small eating episode—it's not your breakfast, lunch or dinner.

Special Concerns for the College Athlete

Weight Issues

Making weight is an issue in some sports, particularly those with weight categories such as wrestling, weightlifting, gymnastics, dancing, and lightweight rowing. Common practices used by some athletes to perform in a lower weight category are often dangerous and counterproductive. Their bodies initially adapt to some of the restrictive dieting, so serious problems may be masked for some time. However, fasting, sweating off pounds, or restricting calories will ultimately decrease endurance, hamper ability to concentrate, and cause a less than optimal performance. In some situations, such practices have contributed to the death of young athletes.

Some athlete's **weight cycle**. They are at one weight for a sport and then add or lose during the off season. It's obviously best to keep up some sort of exercise routine and eat well throughout the year, but many athletes don't do that. You might find yourself in great shape during the season, but as tryouts for a new season start, you're not where you want to be.

Start training early, and have a realistic plan to get back in shape. Avoid dieting or other restrictive eating patterns. Losing weight quickly can cause you to lose muscle as well as fat, and with muscle loss comes decreased strength. Strive for a sensible eating plan that allows a slow weight loss, and start early.

Losing weight for a sport can be the trigger to developing serious eating disorders. As many as 60 percent of college athletes have been considered eating disordered or at risk for developing an eating disorder. Increased pressure to perform and personality traits such as competitiveness, high achievement, and perfectionism enable athletes to excel in their sport, but also place them at higher risk for eating disorders.

Such disorders among athletes can be life threatening (see Chapter 6). If you or a fellow competitor has an eating disorder, seek counseling. Performing in a sport while eating an inadequate diet or purging limits your abilities, puts you at risk for injuries, and can ultimately kill you. These are serious problems that need to be addressed, even if you're a superstar athlete.

Supplements

Athletes also seem to be particularly vulnerable to highly advertised supplements or **ergogenic** aids. The industry knows that every athlete is looking for an extra something to gain a competitive edge. That makes athletes a big target for supplement promotions and other myths (see Chart 9–10).

Although there are hundreds of supplements on the market, few if any have valid scientific studies to support the claims made about them, and deceptive marketing tactics are often used to promote them. Some of these supplements may be safe, just not effective; others may

CHART 9–10

Top Ten Myths about Sports Nutrition

10. **Vitamin supplements provide you with extra energy.**

    Vitamins do not contain calories, nor do they increase your energy. The additional vitamins athletes need they can easily get by eating a reasonable diet that meets their caloric needs.

9. **Drinking during training causes cramps.**

    You must continue to replace fluids as you exercise. Cramps are not caused by fluid intake.

8. **The more protein you eat, the bigger your muscles will be.**

    Training and adequate protein make bigger muscles. More is not better.

7. **Athletes should take salt tablets to replace the sodium they lose.**

    While you lose sodium through sweating, you can replace what's lost by eating salty foods or adding salt to what you eat.

6. **If you're trying to "make weight," it's best to sweat it off.**

    Making weight by sweating can be a dangerous practice and dehydration impairs your ability to perform.

5. **Don't eat before an event.**

    Your body needs fluids and food to help maintain a constant blood sugar level. It's wise to experiment with foods to see just how much you can comfortably eat before competing.

4. **Bee pollen, chromium picolinate, and carnitine can all help improve athletic performance.**

    While some supplements may be perfectly safe to take, there is little evidence to support the wild claims about their ability to improve athletic performance.

3. **Beer is a good thirst quencher.**

    Drinking alcohol in any form is not recommended to replace fluids because alcoholic drinks are dehydrating.

2. **To get the best out of carbohydrate loading, eat a big plate of pasta the night before an event.**

    Carbohydrate loading is accomplished most effectively by altering your training schedule and eating a relatively high-carbohydrate diet throughout training.

1. **Taking supplements is the best way to bulk up.**

    If you need to bulk up, add more food and exercise more. Supplements can't replace food, only supplement it.

not be safe at all. It's easy to get sucked into thinking you need that extra something.

Eating well influences how you feel and how you perform. But if something seems too good to be true, even something supported by a coach or trainer, it's wise to consult an independent, knowledgeable source.

FOR MORE INFORMATION . . .

Books

Clark, N. 2003. *Nancy Clark's Sports Nutrition Guidebook*, 3rd ed. Champaign, Il. Human Kinetics.

Eberle, G. 2000. *Endurance Sports Nutrition.* Champaign, Il. Human Kinetics.

Kleiner, S. *Power Eating*, 2nd. Ed. Champaign, Il. Human Kinetics.

Litt, A. 2004. *Fuel for Young Athletes.*, Champaign, Il. Human Kinetics.

Websites and Organizations

www.SCANdpg.org

www.ncaa.org
Look under 'N" for nutrition information

www.gssiweb.com

www.supplementwatch.com

www.consumerlab.com

Special Requests

Eating on campus can be a challenge for anyone. Tack on the need to follow a special diet, or eat special kinds of foods and the challenge can seem impossible. Worry not. You can make it work, if:

- You know your problem foods
- You understand how to read food labels, and
- You take time to talk with the people who prepare your food.

This chapter isn't about helping you figure out if you have a food-related problem. For that you should check with a health care professional. Instead, this chapter is designed to be a roadmap of sorts, one that guides you in making healthful food choices while you are away from home—one that will help you meet your special diet needs.

Most colleges are ready, willing and able to handle *reasonable* special food requests. However, the ultimate responsibility for eating well is yours. The job of getting what you need, essentially rests in your lap.

Special Diets

There are several different types of diets that college students follow. Some people may have allergies, others may have digestive problems that make it difficult for them to eat certain foods or ingredients and still others may have a condition, such as diabetes, that requires a certain type of meal plan. Below is a brief explanation of some of the more common diets college students may be following and dietary guidelines to help you enjoy eating well on campus.

Note: It is strongly recommended that for any special diet needs, you talk with a registered dietitian. He or she can help you manage your diet more successfully, especially if you are living on your own for the first time.

Food Allergies and Food Intolerances

Often, food allergies and food intolerances are considered one in the same. (See Chart 10–1) These two conditions may involve the same types of food, even cause the same types of reactions, but they happen for different reasons and their reactions in the body can be very different. For successful management of food allergies and intolerances it is important to understand exactly what they are.

Food Allergies

Food allergies occur when the body's immune system reacts abnormally to a food or certain ingredients within a food. The symptoms or problems appear soon after eating. Theoretically, a person can

> ### CHART 10–1
>
> # Allergy or Intolerance?
>
> Are you allergic to milk or do you have a lactose intolerance? There is a difference. People with lactose intolerance have a hard time digesting the sugar in milk called **lactose**. People who are allergic to milk, are not affected by its lactose—instead, they tend to be allergic to the protein in milk. Most lactose intolerance sufferers are able to consume some dairy products, but those with a milk allergy often need to eliminate all milk from their diets. Lactose free products such as Lactaid milk may be helpful to those who are lactose intolerant. In a similar way, people confuse **celiac disease** with a **wheat allergy**. Those with wheat allergy must avoid only wheat-containing products, whereas people with celiac disease must avoid wheat as well as other grains that contain gluten—a protein in wheat, oats, rye and barley.

be allergic to any food, but eight foods tend to be the most frequent offenders. They are: **milk, eggs, wheat, soy, fish, shellfish, peanuts** and other **tree nuts** including **walnut** and **cashews**. While you can certainly be allergic to more than one food, being allergic to several is rare.

Food Intolerances

A food intolerance occurs when the body does not "tolerate" or digest a particular food or substance within a food. Unlike a food allergy, food intolerances do not involve the immune system. The symptoms can occur right after the food is eaten or they may present even days later. This alone can make it difficult to pinpoint exactly which food is the problem.

Food allergies and food intolerances cause reactions in the body—anything from mild symptoms to quite extreme ones. Getting a stuffy nose, a skin rash or hives, becoming nauseated or experiencing diarrhea are all typical reactions. In rare cases, a food allergy will result in a dramatic and potentially life-threatening event called an anaphylactic reaction. Symptoms appear quickly after eating the offending food. The throat may swell, there may be difficulty with breathing

CHART 10–2

How to Work with Campus Food Service

1. Ask campus administration for the name of the food service director in your dining hall.

2. Set up an appointment to meet with the food service manager and dietitian if available.

3. Identify your special diet.

4. Ask for a copy of the menus. (Often there is a 4–5 week cycle.)

5. Identify items you would like to eat and ask the food service director/dietitian to check the recipe, appropriate food labels and food companies selling the food to determine if they are safe for you to eat.

6. Depending on your allergy/sensitivity, determine if there is a special place in the kitchen to keep foods separate to avoid cross contamination concerns.

    Cross contamination occurs when a product you know is free of a particular allergen comes in contact indirectly with the suspected allergen. To avoid cross contamination:

    • Request food service workers use a new pair of gloves before handling your food.

    • Do not use common cutting boards or grills unless they have been wiped clean before using them.

    • Avoid fried foods—often cooking oil is shared amongst several different types of food.

    • Store your special foods in containers labeled with bright stickers.

    • Avoid buffets and salad bars where serving utensils may stray into contaminated products.

    • If having sandwich meats sliced, ask to have the deli slicer cleaned before foods you can eat are cut on the slicer.

    • If having ice cream, ask that a clean scoop be used before dishing up your portion.

    • Consider using your own toaster.

7. Always say thank you to a server who has helped and the food service director who goes out of his or her way to accommodate your requests. A little gratitude goes a long, long way.

and ultimately a person can become unconscious. Should this happen to you, get yourself to the nearest emergency room immediately or call 911.

If you have ever experienced an anaphylactic reaction to a food, you should schedule a meeting with the food service director on campus as soon as you arrive at school. Together you can discuss your food allergy and strategies for avoiding trouble (Chart 10–2). You should be very specific about the food(s) that cause a reaction. You may be advised by your doctor to wear a medical alert bracelet and the dining hall may ask you to carry an "epi" pen with you in the event of an emergency.

If you have a food allergy, you need to completely eliminate the offending food from your diet. If you have a food intolerance, you may be able to eat a small quantity of a troublesome food before you experience symptoms (Chart 10–3). To avoid problems, be vigilant in knowing what you eat and learn how to read food labels. Both strategies will help you stay well and feel good (Chart 10–4).

CHART 10–3

Lactose Content of Foods

FOOD	AMOUNT	LACTOSE (gm)
Milk	1 cup	11
Buttermilk	1 cup	10
Ice milk	½ cup	9
Ice cream	½ cup	6
Yogurt	1 cup	5
Sour cream	½ cup	4
Cottage cheese	½ cup	3
American cheese	1 slice	2
Hard cheese	1 oz.	1
Cream cheese	1 oz	1
Butter	1 Tbs.	Trace

Celiac Disease

Celiac disease, also called celiac sprue or gluten intolerance, is a challenging and serious food intolerance. It is a genetically based autoimmune disease caused by a sensitivity to gluten—a protein found in wheat, rye, and barley. If you have celiac disease, eating gluten triggers an immune response in the body that damages the lining of your small intestine. The fallout can include diarrhea, constipation, weight loss, fatigue and gas. The condition affects the absorption and use of important vitamins and minerals your body needs such as iron, calcium, folic acid and fat soluble vitamins. If left untreated it can result in anemia and bone disease.

Unlike other intolerances, which may allow you to at least eat small amounts of the problem food, people with celiac disease must avoid any food containing gluten. Even a minute amount can wreak havoc (Chart 10–4). Following a strict gluten-free diet allows the intestine to heal and return to its healthful state.

One never outgrows celiac disease. But, many people manage it and manage it quite well (See chart 10–5). Fortunately, there are many grains available to eat that do not contain gluten and there are also a growing number of gluten-free products on the market. In fact, gluten-free foods are considered one of the fastest growing specialty food markets.

When you speak with the dining services director about your diet, bring in a few favorite products to help him or her understand what's available and which products you like. For some directors this may be their first exposure to gluten intolerance. They may not be aware of the possibilities available.

Sulfite Sensitivity

The sulfur-based compounds found in certain foods such as those listed in Chart 10–4 can cause problems for people with a sulfite sensitivity. These compounds occur naturally within a food or they may be added to products as a preservative or flavor enhancer. They are also found in beer and wine.

CHART 10-4

Tips for Food Allergies and Food Intolerances*

Milk allergy: The following words may indicate the presence of milk.

Milk (derivative, powder, protein, solids, malted, condensed, evaporated, dry, sour milk, sour milk solids, whole, lowfat, nonfat, skimmed)	Buttermilk	Lactoglobulin
	Casein	Lactose
	Caseinates	Lactulose
	Cheese	Nougat
	Cream	Pudding
	Curds	Rennet
	Custard	Sour Cream
	Dairy	Whey
	Ghee	Yogurt
Artificial butter flavor	Half & Half	Anything labeled with a "D" or "DE"
Butter, butter fat, butter oil	Kefir	
	Lactalbumin	

Milk may be hidden in the following products:

Baked goods	"non-dairy" substitutes	Pre-breaded foods
Bread	Imitation sour cream	Sherbet
Canned fish	Margarine	Soups
caramel	Luncheon meats, hot dogs, sausage	Sports bars, energy bars, breakfast bars
Chocolate		

Egg allergy: The following words may indicate the presence of eggs

Albumin	Emulsifier	ovomuccoid
Albumen	French Toast	Ovovitellin
Aviden	Globulin	Quiche
apovitellin	Livetin	Sauces (Béarnaise, Hollandaise, Newburg)
Binders	Mayonnaise	
Custard	Meringue	
Egg (dried, powdered, solids, white, yolk)	Ovalbumin	Simplesse
	Ovomucin	Souffles
Eggnog	Ovamucoid	
Egg noodles	Ovoglobulin	

* If you are allergic or intolerant or suspect you may be, you are advised to get complete information about food sources of allergens and not rely on this list. This is just a general guideline to indicate the places these allergens may be found.

Egg may be hidden in the following products

Baked goods	Instant cereals	Root beer
Baking mixes	Lemon curd	Specialty coffee
Candy	Pasta	Tempura
Ice cream		

Egg can be used as a glaze on baked goods to give a glaze

Wheat allergy: The following words may indicate the presence of wheat

Bran	Cracker	Matzoh
Bread	Cracker meal	Semolina
Breadcrumbs	Durum	Spelt
Bulgur	Farina	Triticale
Cereal extract	Flour	Wheat: bran, germ,
Cracker meal	Gluten	malt, starch
Couscous	Graham	Whole wheat

Wheat may be hidden in the following products:

Baked goods	Hydrolyzed vegetable	Processed meats
Baking mixes	protein	Stabilizers
Baking powder	Malt	Soy sauce
Cereals, cereal bars	Meatballs, meatloaf,	Sports bars, energy
Coffee substitutes	pre-made	bars
made with grain	hamburgers	Starch
Flavored coffees & teas	Modified food starch	Tamari
Gelatinized starch	Natural flavoring	Vegetable gum
Hydrolyzed plant	Ovaltine	Vegetable starch
protein	Prebreaded foods	

Soybean allergy: The following words may indicate the presence of soy**

Carob	Protein filler	Soybean
Edame	Shoya sauce	Tamari
Hydrolyzed soy protein	Soy (albumin,	Tempeh
Hydrolyzed vegetable	cheese, flour, grits,	Textured vegetable
protein	ice cream, nuts,	protein
Miso	protein, milk,	Tofu, Tofu-based
Monosodium	sprouts, yogurt)	meats/deli products
glutamate (MSG)	Soy sauce	
Protein extender	Soya	

**Soy oil and soy lecithin are not restricted because it is the soy protein which causes the allergic reaction.

Soy may be hidden in the following products

Baked goods
"Bars" such as energy
　bars, sports bars
Breakfast cereal
Candy
Chinese food
Margarine

Meat alternatives
Powdered meal
　replacements
Salad dressing
Sauces (soy, Asian,
　Worcestershire)
Seasonings

Smoothies
Soup
Stabilizers
Thickeners
Vegetable gums,
　starches

Peanut allergy: The following words may indicate the presence of peanuts

Cold-pressed Peanut
　Oil
Ground Nuts
Marzipan

Mandalona
Mixed nuts
Nougat
Peanut

Peanut butter
Peanut flour

Peanut may be hidden in the following products

Alcohol such as
　frangelico and
　amaretto
Asian foods
Asian sauces and
　flavorings
Bars such as energy
　bars and sports
　bars

Baking mixes
Baked goods
Battered or fried food
Candy
Cereals
Dehydrated soup
Goober peas and nuts
Hydrolyzed plant
　protein (hpp)

Hydrolyzed vegetable
　protein (hvp)
Mortadella
Nut butters
Satay
Soups
Trail mix
Vegetable oil

Nut allergy: The following words may indicate the presence of tree nuts

Almonds
Brazil nuts
Cashews
Chestnuts
Hazelnuts (filberts)
Hickory nuts,

Macadamia nuts
Marzipan
Nougat
Nut butters
Pecans
Pesto

Pine nuts (pignolia nuts)
Pistachios
Pralines
Walnuts

Tree nuts may be hidden in the following products

Alcohol such as
　Frangelico and
　Amaretto
Almond paste
Baked goods

Bars such as energy
　bars and sports
　bars
Candy
Cereals

Chocolate
Nut butters
Trail mix
Walnut oil

Fish/shellfish allergy: The following words may indicate the presence of fish or shellfish

Agar	Caviar	Surimi
All species of fish	Fish oil	Worcestershire sauce
All species of shellfish	Omega-3 fatty acids	
Anchovies	Oyster sauce	
Asian sauces	Roe	

Fish/shellfish may be hidden in the following:

Alginic acid or	Caesar salad	Pasta sauce
alginate	Caesar salad dressing	Pizza
Asian foods	Fried foods	

Gluten sensitivity: The following words may indicate the presence of gluten

Barley	Graham flour	Rye
Bulghur	Kamut	Spelt
Einkorn	Oats†(bran, syrup)	Triticale
Emmer	Malt (extract, flavoring,	Wheat (bran, germ,
Farro	syrup)	starch)

Gluten may be hidden in the following products

Cereal	Hydrolyzed vegetable	Modified food starch
Cereal binding agents	protein (HVP)	Starch
Hydrolyzed plant protein (HPP)		

† There is controversy as to whether Oats are permitted on a gluten-free diet.

Sulfites sensitivity: the following words may indicate the presence of sulfites

Sodium and/or potassium bisulfite	Sodium and/or potassium metabisulfite	Sulfite Sulfur dioxide Sulfurous acid

Sulfites may be hidden in the following foods

Alcoholic beverages	Fruit juice, sparkling	Pickles
Baked goods	fruit juice, cider	Pickled foods/
Candy	Gravies and sauces	sauerkraut
Chips	Guacamole	Rice mixes
Dehydrated, pre-cut or peeled potatoes	Jams/jelly	Soup mixes
Dried fruit (excluding raisins and prunes)	Lemon juice, unfrozen Lime juice, unfrozen	Sugar Trail mix
Fresh or frozen shrimp	Maraschino cherries	Wine vinegar
Frosting	Molasses	
	Olives	

CHART 10–5

Celiac Disease and College
by Christy Woodcock, Student, University of Massachusetts

Heading off to college with Celiac Disease seems like a scary thought. Some people may think it is impossible to have a normal college experience because of our diet. I am writing this article to let you know that it's not impossible, and it's not even painful!!

After choosing the school I wanted to attend I had to figure out how I would deal with Celiac Disease at school. My mom and I made calls to the people in charge of dining services. It took them many weeks to finally have time to talk to us, but when they did they were extremely helpful. We told the head of dining services all about the disease. Luckily she had to deal with a celiac student last year, so she already knew the ropes. We decided that I would set up an appointment to talk about the food in the dining hall when I got to school.

Another thing I had to work out was the storage of my gluten free food, such as bread, pasta, cookies, my own mayo, butter, cream cheese, etc. At my school we had the choice of renting or buying a fridge. Usually people rent one with their roommate, but my parents decided it would be better in the long run if we just bought one. When I found out who my roommate was I talked to her about my situation. I told her she could use the fridge, but I needed to make sure there was enough space for my food. She was incredibly understanding about my situation.

I also bought a set of pots, pans, and plates so that I could cook my own food when there was nothing else I could eat at the dining hall. There are many things I found I needed and didn't have. Some of those necessities are paper and plastic (helps cut down on dish washing) plates, bowls, spoons, forks and knifes. I also found it helpful if they were all microwaveable. I got a note from my doctor so that I could get a room near a kitchen in my dorm. I didn't care about this as much as my mom did, but I thought I would do it to make her less stressed!

Once I got to school I met with the head of dining services. She printed me out a list of EVERY meal or food item they ever serve in the dining hall, and the ingredients of all those things. We decided that sending the menu a week early would give me enough time to figure out what I could have each day. (This may sound like a lot of work, but the menu repeats every couple weeks so you get to know what you can and can't have). She told me what some good choices would be, and what to stay away from. I also had to remind her that I couldn't have things such as soy sauce and modified food starch, so you may have to clue them into detailed gluten

containing ingredients. I sat down later that day and read through all of the
listings circling things I could have and crossing out those I couldn't.

I usually have one or two meals a day at the dining hall and occasionally
cook on my own. One of the girls that lives next to me is Dominican and the
other Puerto Rican. They taught me how to cook Spanish food, lots of which
where gluten free!! I discovered new ways to cook bananas, plantains,
chicken, and rice. It has been a great way to learn about different cultures
and learn new gluten free recipes.

Some days I never eat at the dining hall because they have nothing I
can have (or nothing I like, you get sick of salad!). I go shopping at Bread
and Circus and order food online every couple of weeks. Having a store
that I can easily get to from campus and that has a good selection of gluten
free products has been extremely helpful.

If you are thinking it is going to be impossible let me reassure you that
that it's really not so bad.

A person can develop sulfite sensitivity at any time in his or her life.
No one knows exactly what triggers the sensitivity. Reactions range
from mild to life threatening. Typical symptoms include chest tight-
ness, hives, nausea or anaphylactic shock.

Restaurants may use sulfites during food preparation to prevent the
discoloration of foods, such as cut fruits and vegetables. If you are sensitive to sulfite, be sure to ask staff or your server specific questions
about how foods are prepared.

Sulfites can also be found in some medications. Talk with your pharmacist and health care provider about your need to avoid them in prescribed
or over-the-counter medication. Always read labels carefully.

Digestive Problems

Irritable Bowel Syndrome (IBS) is often called "the misunderstood
disease". People who suffer from IBS may complain of bloating, gas,
diarrhea, constipation, cramping or all of the above. It seems to affect
significantly more women than men—exactly why is unclear.

Unlike food allergies, intolerances and sensitivities, foods do not
cause this condition. However, modifying what and how you eat can
help relieve some of its symptoms.

The diet for IBS relief is based on trial and error. The process is commonly termed an "elimination" diet meaning by systematically ruling out certain foods, those that cause problems can be identified. The foods often thought to make IBS symptoms worse are alcohol, chocolate, caffeine, carbonated drinks, fried foods, high fructose foods and "gassy foods" such as beans, cabbage, broccoli and cucumbers.

Approach the elimination of foods in a slow, organized manner. Keep a diary of the eliminations which work and those that do not. Removing too many foods at once may make you feel better, but you will likely not learn much from the process. You will end up eating a very restrictive diet and never fully know which food(s) is causing the problem.

One of the goals of treatment for IBS is to keep the digestive system "regular". That means eating a fiber rich diet. However, not all fiber is created equal (See Chapter 1). Knowing how the different fibers work in your body and learning when you should eat which type of fiber can mean the difference between having symptoms and being pain free.

Soluble fiber is the fiber found in foods such as oatmeal, rice, pasta, bananas, applesauce and potatoes. For IBS sufferers, soluble fiber is the fiber of choice because it is helpful in normalizing bowel function, relieving both diarrhea and constipation.

Insoluble fiber is found in whole grain bread, whole grain cereals, nuts, popcorn, berries, apples, and many veggies. It is very important for good health, but for people with IBS, a diet high in insoluble fiber can cause pain when eaten.

If you enjoy foods that are rich in insoluble fiber, introduce them carefully into your diet. Always increase your water intake at the same time you eat these high fiber foods and avoid eating foods high in insoluble fiber alone or on an empty stomach

Additional diet strategies for living with IBS are found in Chart 10–6.

Hypoglycemia

The term hypoglycemia means low blood sugar. The medical condition of hypoglycemia is rare, but many people can have the symptoms

CHART 10–6

Diet Strategies for IBS Relief

- Try eating small meals more often
- Know the difference between soluble and insoluble fiber. Do not eat insoluble fiber alone or on an empty stomach

Foods high in soluble fiber: applesauce, barley, bananas, carrots, mangoes, papayas, oatmeal, pasta, noodles, rice, rice cereals, flour tortillas, potatoes, yams, sweet potatoes.

Foods high in insoluble fiber: whole wheat bread, whole wheat cereal, wheat bran, granola, meuslix, seeds, nuts, popcorn, legumes, berries, grapes, raisins, apples, oranges, grapefruit, melons, greens, peas, onions, broccoli, Brussel sprouts, cauliflower, tomatoes, cucumbers, green beans, dates, prunes

- Do not overeat. Stop eating when you've had enough.
- Slow down. Eating too quickly can exacerbate symptoms
- Don't wear tight clothing. Anything tight around your stomach can make you feel worse.
- Don't chew gum since it causes you to swallow too much air and may trigger symptoms.
- You might want to eliminate any drinks or foods that are "frothy" such as cappuccinos and soft serve ice creams. Incorporating air into foods may make bloating worse.
- Try eliminating "bubbles" and carbonation from your diet.
- Try drinking mint tea. It may relax your muscles.

of low blood sugar without having an actual diagnosis of hypoglycemia. The most common symptoms of hypoglycemia include headache, dizziness, fainting, shakiness, light-headedness or feeling hungry all of the time. The symptoms tend to occur if a person does not eat often enough or eats the wrong combination of foods.

The goal in managing the symptoms of hypoglycemia is to stabilize blood sugar levels. When you eat and what you eat will minimize symptoms or at least make them more manageable. Symptoms seem to be better controlled if you eat small frequent meals—i.e. eating

---

CHART 10–7

Meal Pattern for Hypoglycemic Diet

First meal around 10:00 A.M.
Small bagel with butter/cheese/fruit

Lunch around 1:00
Turkey sandwich/vegetable soup/fruit

Afternoon snack around 4:00
Hard cooked egg/whole grain crackers/herbal tea

Dinner
Baked chicken/baked sweet potato/salad/dressing/fruit
Ice cream for dessert

Late-night snack
Peanut butter on graham cracker/milk

---

every three to four hours. Each mini-meal should include a balance of protein, fat and complex carbohydrates (Chart 10–7). Complex carbs such as whole grains, fruits and veggies are absorbed more slowly than simple carbs, such as those found in soda, fruit juice and candy. Because they require minimal digestion, simple carbs can be quickly absorbed into your blood stream causing a spike in blood sugar. This holds true particularly if these foods are eaten alone or on an empty stomach. Other diet modifications for managing hypoglycemia are outlined in Chart 10–8.

CHART 10–8

Guidelines for Living with Hypoglycemia

- Eat at consistent times each day
- Avoid alcohol, caffeine, tobacco and other stimulants since they can make the symptoms worse
- Avoid eating and drinking "simple" sugars such as soda, fruit juice, and candy, especially on an empty stomach
- Try and eat every three hours
- At each meal and snack include a mix of proteins, complex carbs and a bit of fat

Hypertension And Cholesterol-Lowering Diets

An increasing number of college students are plagued with health problems similar to those affecting older adults—specifically having a high blood cholesterol level, high blood pressure or both. They are arriving on campus needing to follow a low cholesterol, low fat and/or low sodium diet.

A promising eating plan known as DASH diet or Dietary Approaches to Stop Hypertension (DASH) is often prescribed to help lower both cholesterol and blood pressure. It is low in harmful fats and sodium, and rich in several nutrients that benefit the body. It is similar to the diet recommendations recently advised in the new Dietary Guidelines. (see chapter 1) For a peek at what's in the DASH diet, see Chart 10-9.

Kosher

Most students opting to follow a Kosher diet have checked out their dining options before arriving on campus. Some schools have complete Kosher dining centers while others combine Kosher dining with vegetarian dining centers thereby keeping meat out of the kitchen. Some schools offer Kosher meals that are pre-packaged and can be reheated and some colleges and universities may even have a Hillel on campus where Kosher meals are served or Kosher restaurants are housed.

Polycystic Ovary Syndrome (PCOS)

Polycystic Ovary Syndrome (PCOS) is an endocrine (hormonally-based) disorder that affects 5 to 10 percent of women of childbearing age. It is characterized by irregular menstrual periods, hirsutism (darkening or coarse hair growth appearing in a "male" pattern on the chest, abs, and groin area), excessive facial hair, male balding patterns, acne and other skin changes.

PCOS can affect women of all ages. Symptoms may vary depending on the age of onset. Almost all women with PCOS experience insulin resistance, which can cause weight gain or make it difficult to lose weight

CHART 10–9

DASH Diet

The DASH eating plan shown below is based on 2,000 calories a day. The number of daily servings in a food group may vary from those listed, depending on your caloric needs. Use this chart to help you plan your menus or take it with you when you go to the store.

FOOD GROUP	DAILY SERVINGS (except as noted)	SERVING SIZES	EXAMPLES AND NOTES	SIGNIFICANCE OF EACH FOOD TO THE DASH EATING PLAN
Grains and grain products	7–8	1 slice bread 1 oz dry cereal* ½ cup cooked rice, pasta or cereal	Whole wheat bread, English muffin, pita bread, bagel, cereals, grits, oatmeal, crackers, pasta, or cereal unsalted pretzels and popcorn	Major sources of energy and fiber
Vegetables	4–5	1 cup raw leafy vegetable ½ cup cooked vegetable 6 oz vegetable juice	Tomatoes, potatoes, carrots, green peas, squash, broccoli, turnip greens, collards, kale, spinach, artichokes, green beans, lima beans, sweet potatoes	Rich sources of potassium, magnesium, and fiber
Fruits	4–5	6 oz fruit juice 1 medium fruit ¼ cup dried fruit ½ cup fresh, frozen, or canned fruit	Apricots, bananas, dates, grapes, oranges, orange juice, grapefruit, grapefruit juice, mangoes, melons, peaches, pineapples, prunes, raisins, strawberries, tangerines	Important sources of potassium, magnesium, and fiber
Lowfat or fat free dairy foods	2–3	8 oz milk 1 cup yogurt 1½ oz cheese	Fat free (skim) or lowfat (1%) milk, fat free or lowfat buttermilk, fat free or lowfat regular or frozen yogurt, lowfat and fat free cheese	Major sources of calcium and protein
Meats, poultry, and fish	2 or less	3 oz cooked meats, poultry, or fish	Select only lean; trim away visible fats; broil, roast, or boil, instead of frying; remove skin from poultry	Rich sources of protein and magnesium
Nuts, seeds, and dry beans	4–5 per week	⅓ cup or 1½ oz nuts 2 Tbsp or ½ oz seeds ½ cup cooked dry beans	Almonds, filberts, mixed nuts, peanuts, walnuts, sunflower seeds, kidney beans, lentils, peas	Rich sources of energy, potassium, magnesium, protein, and fiber
Fats and oils†	2–3	1 tsp soft margarine 1 Tbsp lowfat mayonnaise 2 Tbsp light salad dressing 1 tsp vegetable oil	Soft margarine, lowfat mayonnaise, light salad dressing, vegetable oil (such as olive, corn, canola, or safflower)	DASH has 27 percent of calories as fat, including fat in or added to foods
Sweets	5 per week	1 Tbsp sugar 1 Tbsp jelly or jam ½ oz jelly beans 8 oz lemonade	Maple syrup, sugar, jelly, jam, fruit-flavored gelatin, jelly beans, hard candy, fruit punch, sorbet, ices	Sweets should be low in fat

* Equals ½ – 1¼ cups, depending on cereal type. Check the product's Nutrition Facts Label.

† Fat content changes serving counts for fats and oils: For example, 1 Tbsp of regular salad dressing equals 1 serving; 1 Tbsp of a lowfat dressing equals ½ serving; 1 Tbsp of a fat free dressing equals 0 servings.

(Chart 10–10) Approximately 50 percent of women with PCOS are overweight or obese. College age women with PCOS can be at greater risk for developing an eating disorder because of the weight gain and subsequent dieting that occurs. Many women with PCOS may also suffer from depression. Women with PCOS have a much higher rate of infertility. For many, this is the first clue they have the disease.

CHART 10–10

What Is Insulin Resistance?

Insulin is a hormone secreted by the pancreas. Our bodies need insulin to "unlock" the cells and allow the sugar or glucose from food inside the cells. The cells then use the glucose from food for energy. Insulin resistance occurs when the body does not respond properly to the insulin. As a result, the glucose circulating in the blood stays in the blood instead of entering the cells. The body is unable to use the sugar in the blood and signals the pancreas to send out more insulin believing it is needed. Excess insulin and excess sugar circulate in the blood, which can lead to prediabetes.

Once PCOS is properly diagnosed, it is usually managed through a combination of diet, exercise and medications. The diet modifications vary from individual to individual but may include:

- An emphasis on high fiber foods, including whole grains, whole-grain cereals, fresh and dried fruits, vegetables and legumes.
- Carbohydrate foods balanced appropriately with protein and low fat foods.
- The elimination of all simple carbohydrates found in sweets, sweetened beverages and fruit juice.
- The inclusion of foods rich in Omega-3 fatty acids such as certain types of fish, nuts, seeds such as flaxseed and monounsaturated fats such as olive oil, canola oil and nuts.
- Daily exercise.

If you are diagnosed with PCOS or suspect you have it, you will find it very helpful to work with a registered dietitian on campus to help you better understand specific diet manipulations that can work for you.

Summary

Living with your special diet needs may mean extra work on your end. There are many resources to ease the load and help you find a way to ensure you feel well. If you live on campus, meet with the Food Service Director for your dining hall. If your school employs a registered dietitian, consider making an appointment with him or her, too. He or she may be a great bridge between you and the food service department.

Schools are interested in making sure their students excel. Part of that package is eating well. Use the resources available to make sure you do.

F O R   M O R E   I N F O R M A T I O N   .   .   .

Food Allergies, Intolerances and Sensitivities
www.eatright.org
www.foodallergy.org
www.celiac.org
www.celiac.com
www.glutenfreediet.ca
www.fda.gov

IBS
www.eatright.org
www.eatingforibs.com.

Hypoglycemia
www.eatright.org
www.diabetes.niddk.nih.gov/dm/pubs/hypoglycemia/

DASH diet
www.eatright.org
www.nhlbi.nih.gov/health/public/heart/hbp/dash/

PCOS
www.afterthediet.com
www.eatright.org

11

Alcohol, Drugs and Your Diet

C hances are you know why you shouldn't abuse substances like alcohol or drugs, as well as the legal repercussions associated with using them. Not to worry, this chapter isn't a sermon. Instead, it sticks with the theme of this book—nutrition—and looks at how alcohol, drugs, and other chemical substances, such as nicotine and marijuana, can affect your nutritional status, body, and health. It's no surprise: too much of any of these substances is bad news.

Alcohol

Alcohol is the drug of choice for many college students. While studies suggest that alcohol has some health benefits such as helping your heart and clearing out your arteries, many students drink substantially more than what's considered "healthy" (see Chart 11–1). College students purchase an estimated 430 million gallons of alcoholic beverages, including 4 billion cans of beer, annually. That's a lot of alcohol.

CHART 11–1

Moderate and Binge Drinking

Moderate drinking is defined as not more than:
- One drink per day for women or
- Two drinks per day for men.

A drink is considered to be 12 oz. of beer, 5 oz. of wine, or 1.5 oz. of hard liquor.

Binge drinking is defined as:
- Drinking five or more drinks in a row at one sitting for men and four or more in a row for women.

Weight Gain

Alcohol contains calories—and lots of them. For the calorie-conscious person, drinking delivers a double whammy to the waistline. Not only are there calories in alcohol, but there are calories in the foods you find yourself eating while you drink. A recent study found that people who drank alcohol before a meal ate faster and ate more (one-third more calories) than when they drank water or fruit juice before a meal. Alcohol seems to stimulate the appetite.

Something about drinking triggers eating cues regardless of whether you're hungry. The calories from snacking, plus the calories from alcohol, are considered two of the biggest contributors to weight gain for college students.

Some students try to "bank" their calories if they know a big drinking night is coming. Cutting back on food during the day to "save" calories for drinking can have a devastating effect. You'll see, drinking on an empty stomach is a bad idea.

What happens when you drink?

Your body processes alcohol differently from other foods you eat. In general, food is eaten, digested, then absorbed and transported throughout your body to perform various jobs. Alcohol, on the other hand, isn't broken down and digested. Most of it moves quickly and directly from your stomach or intestines into your bloodstream. The absorption of alcohol is accelerated even more if there's no food in your stomach to slow its way into the bloodstream. When you drink on an empty stomach, you can feel, quite suddenly, the sensation of alcohol "going right to your head." Drinking too much, too fast without food in your system makes you more vulnerable to the serious problems of drinking.

Your blood carries alcohol to every organ in your body. It can reach your brain within seconds. Although alcohol may give you an initial "high," this effect is short-lived. Alcohol is actually a depressant and functions like a narcotic. It slows brain activity, dulls your thinking, interferes with your coordination, and clouds your judgment.

Alcohol also affects the amount of antidiurectic hormone produced by your brain, the hormone responsible for controlling urination. Alcohol depresses its production, which is why people who drink beyond moderation often have to go to the bathroom frequently. This increased urination is also partially responsible for the dry or "cotton" mouth you feel the morning after having a few drinks, and the headache that often accompanies it.

How your body reacts to alcohol is somewhat gender-specific. Women handle alcohol differently from men because women tend to be smaller, and their bodies usually contain a higher proportion of fat and a lower proportion of fluid. Since alcohol moves through body fluid and women have less body fluid, the same amount of alcohol is more concentrated in a woman's blood.

Besides differences in size and body composition men and women both produce an enzyme called alcohol dehydrogenase, which helps clear alcohol from the body. Women make less of this enzyme than men do, which again contributes to the longer time alcohol stays in a woman's body.

The liver is responsible for clearing alcohol out of the body. The concentration of alcohol in your blood, (your **blood alcohol level**), is influenced by how quickly your liver can clear it.

The rate at which alcohol moves out of your body depends on:

- Your size;
- Your metabolism;
- How much alcohol you've had to drink.

Most people need at least an hour to metabolize, or clear, half an ounce of alcohol, approximately the amount found in one beer. That means that, **if you drink two beers in an hour, the alcohol in the beer will stay in your blood for at least two hours**. If you drink more than half an ounce in an hour, the excess alcohol accumulates in your blood, causing an increase in your blood alcohol level and, eventually, intoxication. You can calculate how alcohol effects you at www.rupissed.com.

Drinking Too Much

Drinking too much is an individual thing. What you drink, when you drink it, and your body type all play a role in how your body handles alcohol. Inexperienced drinkers or anyone sensitive to alcohol may become intoxicated faster than you'd expect. Alcohol intoxication or alcohol poisoning occurs when the ingested alcohol has slowed down or depressed the body's vital functions. Slow them down too much, and you become unconscious. In the most extreme cases, alcohol intoxication leads to death.

If you've had too much to drink, there's nothing you can do and nothing you can eat or drink that will help you sober up. Popular remedies such as black coffee or a cold shower may make you think you are more alert, but in reality you're not; your brain is not operating at full capacity. Only time cures intoxication.

Getting drunk carries with it some unpleasant side effects. Extreme thirst is common because alcohol acts like a diuretic and actually pulls water out of your body, leaving you dehydrated. Hours of retching followed by a throbbing headache, nausea and just feeling rotten are

CHART 11–2

Do You Have a Problem?

A number of signs can help you identify a problem in yourself or a friend. If you have a few drinks on the weekend, chances are you're fine. However, if you **need** to have those few drinks, and they become more than a few and more than the weekend, read on. If you answer yes to these questions, help is available (see the resource list at the end of this chapter). If you're concerned about a friend's behavior, confront the friend in private. Don't be afraid of losing a friend. In the end, you may be saving his or her life.

- Have you ever thought you should cut down on your drinking or drug use?
- Are your friends, family, or teachers concerned about your drinking or drug use?
- Do you believe your friends think you're more fun when you drink or use drugs?
- Do you need to drink or use drugs if you go out, go to class, or just relax?
- Do you do things under the influence of alcohol or drugs that you wouldn't normally do?
- Do you feel badly about your drinking or drug use?
- Do you ever lie or try to cover up your use of drugs or alcohol?

typical symptoms the morning after. For many people, the day after is a day lost.

How much is too much?

It may be difficult for you to get a handle on what is considered reasonable to drink. No matter where you turn, there seems to be alcohol, and a lot of it. It becomes difficult to determine what is reasonable, especially since abusers become defensive about their habit (see Chart 11–2). Though far from being an endorsement to drink, Chart 11–3 offers guidelines and suggestions for managing your intake responsibly.

CHART 11–3

Responsible Drinking

- Never drink on an empty stomach.
- Drink slowly. It takes an average of one to two hours to metabolize one beer, one four oz. glass of wine, or one shot of hard liquor.
- If you feel the need to have a drink in your hand, alternate between an alcoholic drink and soda, juice, or other non-alcoholic beverage.
- Dilute your mixed drinks with more club soda, water, or fruit juice.
- Know your limit; tolerance is an individual thing.
- Recognize that your judgement is **always** off when you drink.
- Remember . . . you do not have to drink to fit in.

Caffeine

Caffeine has been around for centuries. Most of us get our caffeine from coffee; however, it's found in several other foods as well (see Chart 11–4). Although we don't think of caffeine as a drug, it is one of sorts. Caffeine is a stimulant, whose job is to "rev up the body." This is precisely why, in this time-pressed world, most people choose to drink it.

Caffeine temporarily increases your ability to focus and concentrate. But if you cross over the line between enough caffeine and too much, you'll know it quickly, and so will probably everyone else around you. You feel anxious, jittery, hyper, and not very focused.

Health Issues

There have been many studies evaluating the effects of caffeine on health. These studies are at best controversial and certainly far from being conclusive. Right now, the party line seems to be that:

- Caffeine may speed up your heart rate, but its effect is temporary.
- Caffeine may raise blood pressure slightly, but cutting back doesn't bring high blood pressure down.

CHART 11–4

Caffeine Content of Common Food

FOOD	SERVING	CAFFEINE (mg)
Grande coffee	16 oz.	550
Tall coffee	12 oz.	375
Short coffee	8 oz.	250
Home-brewed	8 oz.	100
Instant coffee	8 oz.	80
Decaffeinated coffee	8 oz.	5
Coca-Cola	12 oz.	45
Mountain Dew	12 oz.	55
Tea, brewed 3 min.	8 oz.	50
Tea, brewed 1 min.	8 oz.	25
Bottled or instant tea	12 oz.	50
Hot chocolate	8 oz.	5
Chocolate bar	1 oz.	6
Chocolate milk	8 oz.	5
Red Bull	8 oz.	80

- Caffeine does not appear to have much effect on the development of benign breast lumps, but women who reduce their caffeine intake will argue differently.

Some studies report that caffeine has its benefits, such as relieving migraine headaches, enhancing alertness, and improving athletic performance. But like its laundry list of potential problems, these claims are hard to prove or disprove.

Athletic Performance

Some athletes are convinced that caffeine enhances their performance. It may give some people a noticeable jolt of energy. How caffeine boosts athletic performance, however, is unclear. Some believe that caffeine increases fat utilization thereby providing athletes with more energy; however, this has not been proven. Whether caffeine affects you athletically depends on your diet, size, and the type of exercise or activity in which you're involved.

Some athletes find that it makes them more nervous and can cause sleep disturbances. Others experience gastric distress, often at inopportune times. Drinking a caffeine-containing beverage before, during, or shortly after training or performing isn't recommended because of its diuretic, or dehydrating, properties. It can be costly and devastating to your performance on the field and harmful to your recovery afterward because it robs your body of necessary water. Athletes take note—caffeine is considered illegal, in large doses (800 mg), by the International Olympic Committee and the NCAA.

It's a Personal Thing

Your reaction to caffeine is highly individual. What is excessive for some people is moderate for others. Most people develop a tolerance for caffeine that can increase over time. If you're not a habitual user, you may feel a buzz after a single cup of coffee; if you're a five-cup-a-day drinker, you may feel nothing at all.

Ridding your body of caffeine is also an individual process. It takes anywhere from one to seven hours for the body to be free of the caffeine you ingested.

How much is too much?

If you have medical problems such as high blood pressure, stomach ailments, or anxiety, it's best to check out other beverage options because caffeine can exacerbate your symptoms. If caffeine makes you feel uncomfortable and interferes with your sleep or how you function during the day, try one of the many decaffeinated possibilities, including herbal tea, decaffeinated tea and coffee, or hot water with lemon.

Should you decide to cut caffeine out altogether, proceed slowly. If you go cold turkey and cut all caffeine out of your diet, you may experience withdrawal in the form of severe headaches and drowsiness. To decrease these withdrawal symptoms, gradually wean yourself by:

- Mixing decaf coffee with regular coffee;
- Substitute decaffeinated beverages such as decaf coffee and soda for those you typically drink that contain caffeine;

- Brew weaker tea by dunking the tea bag for just a few seconds;
- Drink water.

Nicotine

Most college students are aware of the serious health consequences of smoking, yet it remains an extremely popular habit. Many people begin smoking at an early age and assume they will stop when they feel like it. By the time they reach college, they may be ready to quit. However, the addictive properties of nicotine make it hard to just stop.

The motivation for many who start smoking seems to be smoking's ability to help control weight. In light of the dire health consequences of smoking, there can never be a legitimate reason to smoke. But it's important to understand why weight gain is often a common side effect of quitting smoking.

- Nicotine suppresses appetite.

  Once you quit smoking, you may feel hungrier.

- Food takes the place of cigarettes in times of stress.

  If you relied on cigarettes to calm you when you were nervous or anxious, you may turn to food for the same relaxing effect.

- Food tastes better when you stop smoking.

  Nicotine decreases the sensitivity of your taste buds—quit smoking and food tastes better.

- Nicotine influences your metabolism.

  Studies show nicotine increases metabolism, which means you burn more calories when you smoke. Quitting lowers your metabolism unless you take measures. You can increase your exercise to counter the effects of a slower metabolism, and when you're not smoking, exercise should feel a whole lot easier to do.

CHART 11–5

Substituting for Cigarettes

To satisfy the oral cravings:
- Suck a Sugar Daddy, Blow Pop, Tootsie Roll Pop, hard candy, or olive pit
- Chew sugar-free gum
- Chew on toothpicks or plastic straws

To satisfy the non-oral cravings:
- Squeeze "stressballs"
- Have a doodle pad and pencil handy
- Rub "smooth stones"
- Stretch rubber bands

At the end of a meal:
- Brush your teeth
- Chew gum
- Suck on a breath mint
- Use mouthwash

When drinking or partying:
- Chew gum
- Chew on a toothpick
- Keep a glass of water in your hand

Should you decide to quit, the fear of putting on an average of five extra pounds is tough to swallow. But weight gain is not inevitable. The good news about quitting as a college-age student is that the younger you are, the easier it is for your metabolism to overcome the consequences of weight gain.

To combat weight gain after quitting, understand your smoking pattern. Most smokers are not only addicted to the very powerful nicotine in the cigarettes, but they get used to the habit and rituals around smoking as well. Be prepared to substitute for the oral needs and the non-oral dependence (see Chart 11–5). The minute you decide to quit, your whole body will thank you (see Chart 11–6).

CHART 11–6

Benefits of Quitting

- **Within 20 minutes:** Blood pressure drops to normal. Pulse rate drops to normal. Body temperature of hands, feet increase to normal.

- **Within 8 hours:** Carbon monoxide level in blood drops to normal. Oxygen level in blood increases to normal.

- **Within 24 hours:** Chance of heart attack decreases.

- **Within 48 hours:** Nerve endings start re-growing. Ability to smell and taste is enhanced.

- **Within 72 hours:** Bronchial tubes relax, making breathing easier. Lung capacity increases.

- **2 weeks to 3 months:** Circulation improves. Walking becomes easier. Lung function increases up to 30 percent.

- **1 to 9 months:** Coughing, sinus congestion, fatigue, shortness of breath decrease. Cilia re-grow in lungs, increasing ability to handle mucus, clean the lungs, and reduce infection. Body's overall energy level increases.

- **5 years:** Lung cancer death rate for average smoker (one pack a day) decreases from 137 per 100,000 people to 72 per 100,000.

- **10 years:** Lung cancer death rate for average smoker drops 12 deaths per 100,000-almost to the rate for non-smokers.

- **All benefits go down the drain if you puff just one cigarette a day.**

Source: American Cancer Society

Marijuana

Marijuana does have an impact on your diet. After all, one of the strongest arguments for the medicinal use of marijuana is its **appetite-enhancing** properties. It appears that smoking pot does make you want to eat. What you choose while "under the influence" is probably not a well-balanced meal, but anything available at the time. So, again, you may gain weight by increasing your use of marijuana.

Should you choose to smoke pot, not only are good food choices unlikely while you're stoned, your desire to be active, exercise, and keep your body fit is weaker. All in all, marijuana doesn't help you keep fit or healthy.

Stimulants

Cocaine and amphetamines are classified as stimulants. They create a sense of energy and euphoria, and they tend to decrease your appetite. This seems to be the quality that appeals to college students. But beware: these drugs can be addictive. The more you want, the more you need. As you eat less and use more, you can become malnourished, making it more difficult to ward off any illness.

Stimulants create a much more serious problem, however; they keep your body revved up. This means your blood pressure and heart rate increase and you can eventually have serious problems including seizures, stroke, heart attack, and ultimately, death. If you use stimulants while you exercise, they tend to increase your body's temperature, which can be fatal. As the saying goes, "speed kills."

Ephedrine, the "safe and natural" herbal stimulant found in Ma Huang and other "natural" diet aids, is also a stimulant. It appears to be a fairly weak appetite suppressant, yet it exhibits all of the other dangerous stimulant properties. Because these herbal preparations often lack meaningful product control, the actual amount of the active ingredient could be dangerously close to toxic without your even knowing it. Its "natural" label is no endorsement for its safety or effectiveness.

Diet and Drug Interactions

Taking prescribed medications, or even over-the-counter ones may not seem like much of a nutrition issue, but since these go into your body, along with food, they are. Foods and drugs mingle in many ways:

- Some foods may alter how drugs act in your body.

  Have you ever noticed a medication label that states "take on an empty stomach"? That is because the particular medicine is most likely better absorbed without food. Some antibiotics fall into this category. Other medications should be taken with food, since taking the medication on an empty stomach may irritate the stomach and make you feel miserable.

- Some drugs may alter how food is used in your body.

  Certain medications, like the antibiotic tetracycline, may bind with the calcium found in dairy, making both the nutrient and the medicine unusable by your body.

- Drugs and alcohol never mix.

  Sometimes alcohol interferes with how a drug is supposed to work in your body, other times it may increase the intensity of the drug. Either way, the results can be scary and even life-threatening.

It's impossible to know all of the potential interactions that may occur, so remember to read labels carefully. If in doubt, talk to a knowledgeable health care provider such as a pharmacist or doctor

---

CHART 11–7

Food and Drug Interactions

MEDICINE	TAKE WITH FOOD	TAKE ON EMPTY STOMACH	OTHER
Amoxicillin	+++		
Aspirin	+++		
Augmentin	+++		
Biaxin	+++		
Diuretics			Increase potassium-rich food
Erythromycin		+++	
Flagyl	+++		
Ibuprofen	+++		
Oral contraceptives			May need B suppplements
Plendil			Avoid grapefruit juice
Procardia			Avoid grapefruit juice
Tagamet			May need B12 supplement
Tetracycline		+++	Avoid dairy
Zithromax		+++	

(see Chart 11–7).

This is by no means an exhaustive discussion of substance use and abuse. At the very least, it should be an eye-opener. Just about everything you put in your body has the potential to affect your nutritional status and certainly your health. You're not only what you eat, but also what you drink, smoke, inhale, and swallow.

FOR MORE INFORMATION . . .

Books

Donkersloot, M. and L.H. Ferry. 1999. *The How to Quit Smoking and Not Gain Weight Cookbook.* New York: Three Rivers Press.
Katahn, M. 1994. *How To Quit Smoking Without Gaining Weight.* New York: W.W. Norton.

Resources

Beer, Booze, & Books.
http://www.beerboozebooks.com

Students Against Drugs and Alcohol.
http://www.sada.org

PART IV
College Cooking

12

Equipping Your Kitchen

Great-tasting meals can certainly be prepared in a gourmet kitchen, but they can also be prepared in your dorm room. No question about it, a spacious, well-outfitted kitchen is a bonus, but it won't necessarily make you a better cook. What you need is a little creativity, a few gadgets, some standard ingredients, and several reliable recipes to produce everything from simple lunches to elaborate dinners.

A Tour of Your Kitchen: Major Appliances

If you're well acquainted with the kitchen, you may want to skip this section; however, if you consider yourself "appliance-challenged," read on. What follows is a quick tour of your basic kitchen, which in turn will help you figure out how best to set up a makeshift kitchen area in your dorm room or a full-sized kitchen in your apartment or group home.

Refrigerators: What Goes in Them

Most colleges and universities will rent you a small refrigerator. A refrigerator is where you store **all perishables**—any food that spoils and becomes inedible without refrigeration. Typical perishables include:

- Milk
- Yogurt
- Eggs
- Tofu
- Butter

Fruit and veggies last longer if stored in a refrigerator, but they can be left on a cool windowsill for several days. Some foods such as mayonnaise, mustard, and catsup can be stored on a shelf, but require refrigeration after they are opened. The label on a container will tell you if it requires refrigeration after opening, so get in the habit of reading labels carefully.

Refrigerators: What Comes Out

Refrigerators work best when they're not overpacked. An over-stuffed refrigerator may not keep foods at a safe temperature—40 degrees or less. Conversely, refrigerators can get too cold. When this happens, food begins to freeze, and, although it's still safe to eat, it may not taste quite right. Food can't be stored indefinitely in the refrigerator. Strange, inedible, and possibly harmful life grows on food that has been kept too long (see Chart 12–1).

The Freezer

The refrigerator's smaller, colder compartment is the freezer. If you're lucky enough to have a larger-sized freezer, you will have room

CHART 12–1

Keeping Food Safe

PRODUCT	REFRIGERATOR (40° F)	FREEZER (0°F)
Eggs		
Fresh, in shell	3 weeks	Don't freeze
Raw yolks, whites	2–4 days	1 year
Hardcooked	1 week	Don't freeze well
Liquid pasteurized eggs or egg substitutes, opened	3 days	Don't freeze
unopened	10 days	1 year
Mayonnaise, commercial Refrigerate after opening	2 months	Don't freeze
TV Dinners, Frozen Casseroles Keep frozen until ready to serve		3–4 months
Deli & Vacuum–Packed Products		
Store-prepared (or homemade) egg, chicken, tuna, ham, macaroni salads	3–5 days	These products don't freeze well.
Pre-stuffed pork & lamb chops, chicken breasts stuffed with dressing	1 day	These products don't freeze well.
Store-cooked convenience meals	1–2 days	These products don't freeze well.
Commercial brand vacuum-packed dinners with USDA seal	2 weeks, unopened	These products don't freeze well.
Soups & Stews		
Vegetable or meat-added	3–4 days	2–3 months
Hamburger, Ground & Stew Meats		
Hamburger & stew meats	1–2 days	3–4 months
Ground turkey, veal, pork, lamb & mixtures of them	1–2 days	3–4 months

PRODUCT	REFRIGERATOR (40° F)	FREEZER (0°F)
Hotdogs & Lunch Meats		
Hotdogs, opened package	1 week	In freezer wrap, 1–2 months
unopened package	2 weeks	In freezer wrap, 1–2 months
Lunch meats, opened	3–5 days	In freezer wrap, 1–2 months
unopened	2 weeks	In freezer wrap, 1–2 months
Bacon & Sausage		
Bacon	7 days	1 month
Sausage, raw from pork, beef, turkey	1–2 days	1–2 months
Smoked breakfast links, patties	7 days	1–2 months
Hard sausage—pepperoni, jerky sticks	2–3 weeks	1–2 months
Ham, Corned Beef		
Corned beef		
In pouch with pickling juices	5–7 days	Drained, wrapped 1 month
Ham, canned Label says keep refrigerated	6–9 months	Don't freeze
Ham, fully cooked—whole	7 days	1–2 months
Ham, fully cooked—half	3–5 days	1–2 months
Ham, fully cooked—slices	3–4 days	1–2 months
Fresh meat		
Steaks, beef	3–5 days	6–12 months
Chops, pork	3–5 days	4–6 months
Chops, lamb	3–5 days	6–9 months
Roasts, beef	3–5 days	6–12 months
Roasts, lamb	3–5 days	6–9 months
Roasts, pork & veal	3–5 days	4–6 months
Variety meats—Tongue, brain, kidneys, liver, heart, chitterlings	1–2 days	3–4 months

PRODUCT	REFRIGERATOR (40° F)	FREEZER (0°F)
Meat Leftovers		
Cooked meat and meat dishes	3–4 days	2–3 months
Gravy and meat broth	1–2 days	2–3 months
Fresh Poultry		
Chicken or turkey, whole	1–2 days	1 year
Chicken or turkey pieces	1–2 days	9 months
Giblets	1–2 days	3–4 months
Cooked Poultry, Leftover		
Fried chicken	3–4 days	4 months
Cooked poultry dishes	3–4 days	4–6 months
Pieces, plain	3–4 days	4 months
Pieces covered with broth, gravy	1–2 days	6 months
Chicken nuggets, patties	1–2 days	1–3 months

Source: United States Department of Agriculture.

to keep ice cream, frozen meals, pizza, and veggies. If it's much smaller, you need to pick carefully—maybe frozen vegetables and some ice pops.

If you buy meat, chicken, or fish and don't plan to eat it within a day or two, it should be stored in the freezer. Since most of your cooking will probably be for one or two people, separate the meat you buy into small portions and rewrap them before freezing. Then you can **defrost** or thaw only the amount of food you need.

The optimum **temperature of a freezer is 0 degrees**. You might not have a thermometer inside your refrigerator/freezer, so pay close attention to how solid the food in the freezer feels. If ice cream gets too soft or the water in ice cube trays won't freeze, your freezer isn't working properly. Foods stored in a freezer that is too warm may be unsafe to eat.

Once meat or frozen foods have thawed, they need to be cooked and eaten within two days. Don't refreeze them if they have reached room temperature because at room temperature harmful bacteria multiply

CHART 12–2

What Is Food Poisoning?

Food poisoning, or as it is technically called, food-borne illness, is caused by eating food that has been contaminated in some way by bacteria, mold, viruses, or parasites. This contamination can occur when:

- The food comes in contact with a food handler who is carrying some bacteria. For instance, if a waiter who is sick accidentally sneezes on the food before it's served to you, that food can potentially carry something that can make you sick when you eat it.

- Raw food can carry bacteria, which may be completely safe once it is cooked. However, if the raw food comes in contact with the food you're eating and that bacteria is transferred, you can become ill. For instance, if a knife is used to cut a piece of raw chicken and is then used to chop carrots, the bacteria can be transferred to the carrots.

- Food that is kept at temperatures that promote growth of bacteria is then eaten. For instance, if a chicken casserole is left out on a counter for several hours before you eat it, you could become sick from bacteria that has been allowed to grow.

Food-borne illness sometimes feels just like the flu. You may have diarrhea, feel fatigued, and have a stomachache, headache, or fever. These symptoms can hit you anytime from 30 minutes to two weeks after eating infected food. Most symptoms pass within 24 to 48 hours. You should always call a doctor if:

- You have bloody diarrhea;
- You are vomiting or have very bad diarrhea, which could lead to dehydration if not treated;
- You have a stiff neck, fever, and headache; or
- The symptoms last longer than three days.

CHART 12–3

Keep or Toss?

1. I defrosted chicken breasts, but don't want to use them now. Can I refreeze them?
2. There's mold on my cheese. Is it safe to eat?
3. If a food smells bad, is it safe to eat?
4. Should I use a wood or plastic cutting board?
5. If I marinate meat, can I use the marinade as a sauce?

Answers

1. If you defrost food in the refrigerator, not on the counter or in the microwave, it's safe to refreeze them.
2. If it's hard cheese, you can trim away the mold and eat the cheese. However, if the mold is on cottage cheese, cream cheese, other "soft cheese", or other foods, they should not be eaten.
3. Generally, food that smells bad probably will taste bad. However, most contaminated foods don't look or smell bad.
4. Since bacteria can fit itself nicely into the grooves on a wood board, it's better to use plastic when cutting raw meat, poultry, or fish. However, it's always a good idea to have two boards and label one to be used only for the above items. Always wash all boards after each use with hot, soapy water.
5. Marinades can only be used if they have been thoroughly cooked.

---

quickly. The food may look perfectly fine, but don't take any chances. You may feel like you're throwing out good money, but you won't be jeopardizing your health. Food poisoning can be a very unpleasant and, in some cases, a serious condition (see Charts 12–2 and 12–3). Keep this in mind when you pack for your next picnic or tailgate party (see Chart 12–4).

Stove, Oven, and Toaster Ovens

These appliances cook your food. If you live in an apartment, you'll have a stove—the top of it is called the cooktop or range and the bottom is the oven. The cooktop contains the burners, which run on electricity or gas. You use the:

- **Cook top** to boil, simmer, stew, poach, and sauté;

CHART 12–4

Packing a Safe Picnic (or Tailgate Party!)

1. Wash hands before and after preparing food.
2. Pack food in a well insulated container. By ice or icepacks to keep temperatures below 40° F.
3. If you are grilling, keep raw meats and ready-to-eat foods separate.
4. Seal raw or thawed meats in heavy plastic wrap to prevent juices from contaminating other foods.
5. When grilling, remove from the cooler only the amount of raw meat, fish or poultry that will fit on the grill at one time.
6. If you are marinating meat or chicken, don't reuse marinade.
7. Throw away perishable items. Foods should not be left unrefrigerated for more than two hours. In hot weather (90° or above) this time is reduced to one hour.
8. Keep hot food hot and keep cold food cold.
9. During the summer, transport the cooler in the back seat of your air-conditioned car instead of in your hot trunk.
10. Pack moist towelettes to clean.

- **Oven** to bake, roast;
- **Broiler**, or top shelf of an electric oven, to broil or grill.

In a gas oven, the broiler may be located in a drawer under the oven. A toaster oven, although much smaller, will do the same kinds of cooking as a larger oven, just in smaller quantities.

Microwave Oven

If you've grown up with a microwave oven in your kitchen at home, chances are it was used mainly for cooking frozen entrées or reheating or "nuking" cooked foods. If you are in a dorm and only have a microwave oven and no other appliances, it can be used for all of your cooking. The recipes in Chapter 14 list specific instructions for preparing foods in a microwave.

Microwave foods should be cooked only in containers specifically designed for the microwave. Cooking foods in margarine containers, other plastic containers, and certain pottery may cause chemicals from the container to leach out into your food, some of which may be linked to increased risk for cancer. Check to make sure your dishes are microwave-safe. Since microwaves are reflected by metal, cooking in a microwave oven with metal or aluminum foil will damage the oven. Only use foil if the directions specifically state it is safe to be cooked in a microwave oven.

Microwave ovens don't heat food evenly. Cooked foods can be extremely hot in one area and stone cold in another, so stir the food thoroughly after it's been cooked. Because heat builds up in microwave foods, never put your face or hands near the dish when you uncover it, and always use a potholder when removing food from the microwave oven.

Essential Equipment, Tools, and Gadgets

There are necessities for any kitchen, no matter what its size (see Chart 12–5). Kitchen equipment comes in all price ranges. Purchase the best you can afford when it comes to knives, pots, and pans. Better-quality pots and pans allow food to cook more evenly. Better, sharper knives are easier to use and a whole lot safer. For nearly everything else such as plates, glassware, measuring tools, etc., quality isn't as important. If you can plan ahead, shop garage sales to pick up what you need.

Shopping for Food

Where you actually purchase your food may be a bit tricky. Many campus bookstores sell basic supplies; however, you pay a premium price for convenience. Some schools have a scaled-down grocery store right on campus, but again prices may be steep. To get a better deal, you may have to go off campus to a real supermarket. The hassle factor and the cab fare may be worth it when you consider the better selection of food and more competitive prices.

CHART 12–5

Kitchen Essentials

For the dorm room

- 2 microwave-safe mixing bowls, 1 large and 1 small
- 9"x 9" baking dish
- 2 sharp knives, 1 paring knife, and 1 larger knife for chopping, dicing, etc.
- Liquid and dry measuring cups
- Measuring spoons
- Small cutting board
- 1 wooden spoon
- 1 rubber spatula
- Can opener
- Bottle opener
- Small hand grater or electric chopper
- Aluminum foil
- Plastic wrap
- Ziplock bags
- Sponge
- Colander
- Paper towels, paper plates, napkins, plastic utensils
- Potholder

For the full-size kitchen

Add to the above items:

- 10" non-stick fry pan
- 2 or 3 quart saucepan
- Vegetable steamer
- Toaster oven
- Dishes, glasses, silverware

Nice to have, but not essential

- Toaster oven
- Tea kettle
- Coffee maker
- Garlic press
- Muffin tins, loaf pans, cake pans
- Blender or food processor
- George Foreman's Lean Mean Grilling Machine

There is a psychology to how supermarkets are set up. They're geared to sell you more than you need. The most widely advertised foods are at eye level on the shelves. They tend to be the most expensive, too. **Look high and low, literally, to get the best variety and best-priced products**. Be aware of the setup in a supermarket that encourages impulse buying. Popular items are often placed at the ends of aisles or at the cash registers, implying "sale." Sometimes these are items on sale, sometimes they're not.

Rule number one to supermarket shopping is—go to the market prepared. That means with:

- A list in hand;
- Food in your stomach.

Without a list you tend to forget what you need and what you don't. You can end up wasting time and money. Shopping when you're hungry makes any food look good—translation: wasted money and food you probably don't need.

Larger stores will have "name brands"—e.g., Breyer's ice cream, Campbell's soup, and "store brands"—generics. Store brands are generally less expensive. Use unit pricing to comparison shop (see Chart 12–6). Some items are discounted when you buy them in volume. Some are not. If you're cooking for one or two, large-volume purchases may actually cost you more because you end up throwing some food out. Bulk shopping (scooping food out of bins) can be a good bet. It allows you to take the amount you know you can use, and it's often less expensive than packaged food. Large chains and co-ops often have great bulk shopping sections.

CHART 12–6

Unit Pricing

It's easy to compare prices between two similar items that are available in different sizes by using the unit price label affixed to the supermarket shelf directly under the product being sold.

BRAND TOMATO SAUCE 12 oz.

YOU PAY

$2.99

UNIT PRICE

11.7¢

PER OUNCE

GENERIC TOMATO SAUCE 15 oz.

YOU PAY

$1.99

UNIT PRICE

8¢

PER OUNCE

Food Labels

More than 90 percent of processed and packaged foods carry a standardized food label. Learning how to read the label (see Chart 12–7) enables you to get the best nutritional value in your food. Not every food has to be a nutritional superstar, but by reading food labels, you can pick out many that are.

Many food packages also have an **expiration date**. That tells you when a food should no longer be eaten because it may be spoiled. There is also a **sell by date** on foods. Grocery stores are supposed to pull products from their shelves once this date passes; however, food may still be edible for up to a week past the sell by date. Pay close attention to food dating. Quality, taste, nutritional content, and safety of a product can change once this date passes.

Buying Fruits and Vegetables

Produce (fruits and vegetables) is the first section in a supermarket. Produce ranks high on the nutrition meter, but is lacking in many college students' diets. Fruits and vegetables can be expensive, they spoil quickly, and some are not very portable if you're on the go most of the time. Buy only what you know you can use in one week. Inspect the produce before you buy it, and avoid foods that are bruised or have bad spots (see Chart 12–8).

Remove the obstacles to eating lots of fruits and veggies because they make a big difference in your energy level, the strength of your immune system, and the health of every cell in your body. Chart 12–9 points out ways to maximize your fruit and veggie intake.

If you can't go food shopping often, buy frozen or canned produce to supplement the fresh. It's more economical to buy frozen foods in bags than boxes. Use the portion you need from the bag and retie the bag to keep them fresh.

Plain, non-sauced, frozen vegetables are nutritionally similar to fresh vegetables and will last for months rather than days. Canned vegetables may be higher in sodium and slightly lower in nutrients, but even they're better than ignoring the group altogether. Canned fruit, packed in its own juice, is quite nutritious and can supplement your diet when fresh fruit is hard to come by.

Buying Poultry, Meat, and Fish

The fresh meat case in a large supermarket has many cuts of meat and poultry. The easiest, although not the most economical, way to purchase poultry is to buy it already cut up in pieces. Even easier are boneless, skinless chicken breasts. They are versatile and can be used in many dishes.

Beef is sold in a variety of cuts and grades. **Prime** meat is the most tender and most expensive, followed by **choice**. The cut of beef is specific for how you plan to cook it. Steaks, chops, and roasts are tender and should be cooked with dry heat, such as broiling, grilling, and roasting. Stew beef, because it's generally a tougher cut, needs to be cooked by stewing in liquid for a few hours. Chopped or ground beef can be prepared using a variety of cooking techniques, including broiling, stir-frying, and baking. Fish can be purchased fresh, frozen, or canned. If it's fresh, it should have no smell to it, and once purchased, should be eaten within a day or two. If fresh is unavailable, frozen fish will do just fine in most recipes. Canned tuna packed in water and canned salmon both offer a lot of the nutritional benefits found in fresh or frozen fish, and they can be used in many recipes.

Buying Dairy Products and Eggs

In the dairy section, look closely for the sell by dates on milk, yogurt, cottage cheese, etc. Products should be good for one week after a sell by date. Check packages of cheese for mold—some stores stock new products on top of older products or don't turn products over fast enough to keep the stock fresh. Expired dates are not that uncommon.

When purchasing eggs, open the carton and look for any cracked ones. They're an invitation for salmonella poisoning, so don't purchase a carton if it contains a cracked egg. (And if you've accidentally purchased a carton with a cracked egg, don't use it.) Check egg containers for freshness dating as well.

CHART 12–7

Reading Food Labels

The Nutrition Facts Label—An Overview:*

The information in the main or top section (see #1–4 and #6 on the sample nutrition label below), can vary with each food product; it contains product-specific information (serving size, calories, and nutrient information). The bottom part (see #5 on the sample label below) contains a footnote with Daily Values (DVs) for 2,000 and 2,500 calorie diets. This footnote provides recommended dietary information for important nutrients, including fats, sodium and fiber. The footnote is found only on larger packages and does not change from product to product.

① **Start Here**

② **Check Calories**

③ **Limit these Nutrients**

④ **Get Enough of these Nutrients**

⑤ **Footnote**

Nutrition Facts

Serving Si e 1 cup (228g)
Servings Per Container   2

Amount per Serving

Calories 250   Calories from Fat 110

	% Daily Value
Total Fat 12g	18%
Saturated Fat 3g	15%
Trans Fat 3g	
Cholestrol 30mg	10%
Sodium 470mg	20%
Total Carbohydrate 31g	10%
Dietary Fiber 0g	0%
Sugars 5g	
Protein 5g	

Vitamin A	5%
Vitamin C	2%
Calcium	20%
Iron	4%

Percent Daily Values are based on a 2,000 calorie diet.
Your Daily Values may be higher or lower depending on your calorie needs.

	Calories	2,000	2,500
Total Fat	Less than	65g	80g
Sat Fat	Less than	20g	25g
Cholestrol	Less than	300mg	300mg
Sodium	Less than	2,400mg	2,400mg
Total Carbohydrate		300g	375g
Dietary Fiber		25g	30g

⑥ **% Daily Value**

5% or Less
is Low

20% or More
is High

* For more information, go to http://www.cfsan.fda.gov/~dms/fdnewlab.html

Nutrition claims

The government defines the following key words and health claims that appear on labels as follows:

- **Free:** a product contains no amount of, or only trivial or "physiologically inconsequential" amounts of, one or more of these components: fat, saturated fat, cholesterol, sodium, sugars, and calories. For example, "calorie-free" means fewer than 5 calories per serving, and "sugar-free" and "fat-free" both mean less than 0.5 g per serving.
- **Low:** This term can be used on foods that can be eaten frequently without exceeding dietary guidelines for one or more of these components: fat, saturated fat, cholesterol, sodium, and calories.
  - **Low-fat**: 3 g or less per serving
  - **Low-saturated fat**: 1 g or less per serving
  - **Low-sodium**: 140 mg or less per serving
  - **Very low sodium**: 35 mg or less per serving
  - **Low-cholesterol**: 20 mg or less and 2 g or less of saturated fat per serving
  - **Low-calorie**: 40 calories or less per serving.
  - **Low carb** has not been defined by FDA at this point.
- **High**. This term can be used if the food contains 20 percent or more of the Daily Value for a particular nutrient in a serving.
- **Good source**. This term means that one serving of a food contains 10 to 19 percent of the Daily Value for a particular nutrient.
- **Reduced**. This term means that a nutritionally altered product contains at least 25 percent less of a nutrient or of calories than the regular, or reference, product. However, a reduced claim can't be made on a product if its reference food already meets the requirement for a "low" claim.
- **Less**. This term means that a food, whether altered or not, contains 25 percent less of a nutrient or of calories than the reference food. For example, pretzels that have 25 percent less fat than potato chips could carry a "less" claim. "Fewer" is an acceptable synonym.
- **Light**. This descriptor can mean two things:
  - First, that a nutritionally altered product contains one-third fewer calories or half the fat of the reference food. If the food derives 50 percent or more of its calories from fat, the reduction must be 50 percent of the fat.
  - Second, that the sodium content of a low-calorie, low-fat food has been reduced by 50 percent. In addition, "light in sodium" may be used on food in which the sodium content has been reduced by at least 50 percent.
    The term "light" still can be used to describe such properties as texture and color, as long as the label explains the intent–for example, "light brown sugar" and "light and fluffy."
- **Healthy.** A "healthy" food must be low in fat and saturated fat, contain limited amounts of cholesterol and sodium and must provide at least 10 percent of one or more of vitamins A or C, iron, calcium, protein, or fiber. Exempt from this "10-percent" rule are certain raw, canned and frozen fruits and vegetables and certain cereal-grain products.

CHART 12–8

Buying and Storing Fresh Fruits and Vegetables

	LOOK FOR	AVOID	AT HOME
Apples	Firm, crisp, rich color	Bruised or soft spots	Refrigerate
Bananas	Firm, bright yellow	Bruised, dull	Store at room temperature
Broccoli	Dark green with compact clusters	Wilted, clusters open	Refrigerate
Cantaloupe	Rough skin, sweet odor, slightly flexible when pressed	Hard or with moldy spots	Room temperature, refrigerate after cutting
Carrots	Firm, deep orange	Soft, flabby	Refrigerate
Cauliflower	White, compact	Discoloration	Refrigerate
Cucumbers	Heavy for size	Mushy, yellow	Refrigerate
Grapefruit	Heavy for size	Soft, dull color	Store at room temperature or refrigerate
Grapes	Firmly attached to stem	Soft, moldy	Refrigerate; must be completely dry
Honeydew	Slightly soft at end, creamy-colored skin	Bruised	Room temperature until ripe, then refrigerate
Lemons	Firm, rich yellow color	Dull, dark yellow, shriveled skin	Refrigerate
Lettuce Romaine Other leaf	Crisp leaves, bright color Tender leaves	Wilting, discoloration	Refrigerate in plastic bag; must be completely dry
Mushrooms	Closed caps around stem, gills ("tissue" under cap) should be light in color	Dark, discolored gills	Refrigerate in bag or plastic container
Nectarines	Bright color, plump, hard, will ripen	Overly soft, dull	Ripen at room temperature, then refrigerate
Onions	Hard, dry	Blemished	Cool, dark place
Oranges	Firm, heavy, smooth skin	Very light or rough skin	Room temperature for 1 week, refrigerate if kept longer
Peaches	Firm, but soft to the touch	Green color, hard, very soft, bruised	Ripen at room temperature, then refrigerate

Pears	Firm, but not too hard	Wilted or shriveled skin, spots	Ripen at room temperature, then refrigerate
Peppers	Firm, deep color	Flimsy or signs of decay	Refrigerate
Plums	Firm or slightly soft	Too hard or too soft	Ripen at room temperature, then refrigerate
Potatoes	Smooth, firm	Soft spots, bruises, sprouted	Cool, dark place
Strawberries	Firm, red berries with caps attached	Soft, moldy	Refrigerate; must be completely dry
Spinach	Dark green leaves	Wilted	Refrigerate
Squash			
Summer	Glossy outside, tender	Discoloration	Refrigerate
Winter	Heavy for size	Bruised or moldy	Cool, dark place
Sweet potatoes	Firm, smooth, tapered at ends	Worm holes, discoloration	Cool, dark place
Tomatoes	Smooth, red color	Mushy	Refrigerate only when fully ripened

Buying Bread Products and Bakery Items

Bread products are delicious when fresh. They are quite perishable and last less than a week at room temperature, so it's wise to store them in the refrigerator. If you buy a dozen bagels at a time, slice and freeze them. Croissants, donuts, and Danish are all available at the grocery, too. However, they don't contribute much nutritionally, so they're best reserved for special occasions.

Buying Deli and Prepared Foods

If you want to make your own sandwiches, stop by the deli counter. Sliced meats such as ham, turkey, and roast beef won't last more than a few days, so buy wisely. Once at home, rewrap in plastic wrap and store in the refrigerator to keep them fresh.

CHART 12–9
Strive for Five

Five ways to get more fruits and veggies in your life:
- Buy fresh fruits and vegetables when they're in season. Use frozen or canned at other times.
- Keep fruits and veggies user-friendly. Buy pre-washed and cut fresh veggies from the salad bar at the supermarket.
- Try drinking vegetable juice a few times a week.
- Have a fruit or vegetable at each meal.
- Vegetable soup is a perfect snack; try having some soup a few times a week.

Frozen entrées such as TV dinners, and "boxed" meals such as Hamburger Helper can get expensive and are not very satisfying. A steady diet of these will offer you less than optimum nutrition. As an occasional meal, however, they can be fine.

"Foods to go" in the grocery store are an increasingly popular alternative to eating out. Rotisserie chickens to entire meals can be purchased, but almost at restaurant prices. If you go that route, buy the main course, then fix your own potato, salad, or veggies.

Stocking the Kitchen

Charts 12–10 and 12–11 are guides for foods to have on hand for cooking in dorm rooms and full-size kitchens. Survey your space and assess how ready you are to prepare meals. Then, with your list in hand (see Chart 12–12) and food in your stomach, head to the market to get the basics. Before you know it, you might actually eat better, cheaper, and more hassle-free.

CHART 12–10

Staples for Dorm Room and Other Non-Kitchen Cooking

Refrigerator Basics (for small, dorm room-size refrigerator)
- Eggs
- Light or regular butter
- Plain and flavored yogurt
- Skim milk
- Flour or corn tortillas
- Pre-shredded cheese
- Cottage cheese
- Pre-grated Parmesan cheese
- Baby carrots
- Fruit, as space permits

Freezer Staples (for small, dorm room-size freezer)
- Broccoli florets
- Peas
- Chopped spinach

Grains
- Boxed pasta
- Brown or white rice
- Dry cereal
- Instant cooked cereal packets
- Bagels/bread/English muffins

Canned and packaged food
- Chicken and vegetable broth
- Vegetarian refried beans
- Water-packed tuna fish
- Dehydrated soups (Fantastic Foods, Nile Spice, Knorrs)
- Canned soup: minestrone, lentil, vegetable, etc.
- Applesauce
- Plain microwave popcorn

Bottled or jarred food
- Olive oil
- Lemon juice
- Balsamic or red wine vinegar
- Salsa
- Soy sauce
- Mustard
- Low-fat mayonnaise
- Barbecue sauce
- Spaghetti sauce
- Peanut butter
- Jelly

Spices and Seasonings
- Salt and pepper
- Garlic powder, onion salt, celery salt
- Sugar

Other Stuff (space providing)
- Teabags
- Coffee
- Snack foods

CHART 12–11

Stocking the Full Kitchen

Refrigerator Staples

- Eggs
- Light or regular butter
- Light or regular cream cheese
- Plain and flavored yogurt
- Skim milk
- Fresh garlic or jarred minced garlic
- Flour or corn tortillas
- Pre-shredded cheddar or mozzarella cheese
- Cottage cheese
- Pre-grated Parmesan cheese
- Lemon (or lemon juice)
- Vegetables and fruits as space permits

Freezer items

- Bags of frozen broccoli, peas, corn, and other vegetables
- Chopped spinach
- Vegetarian burgers

Grains

- Boxed pasta
- Brown or white rice
- Couscous
- Dry cereal
- Instant cooked cereal packets
- Bread, bagels, pita, or English muffins
- Pizza shell

Canned and packaged foods

- Canned chicken and vegetable broth
- Canned tomatoes
- Tomato sauce
- Tomato paste
- Tomato or vegetable juice
- Vegetarian refried beans
- Canned beans: garbanzo, kidney, black
- Water-packed tuna fish
- Artichoke hearts packed in water
- Water chestnuts
- Dehydrated soups (Fantastic Food, Nile Spice, Knorrs)
- Crushed pineapple in its own juice
- Mandarin oranges in juice
- Raisins
- Applesauce
- Plain microwave popcorn

Bottled or jarred food

- Olive or canola oil
- Balsamic or red wine vinegar
- Salsa
- Soy sauce
- Mustard
- Low-fat mayonnaise
- Barbecue sauce
- Spaghetti sauce
- Apricot jam
- Jelly
- Roasted red peppers
- Peanut butter
- Olives
- Capers

Spices, seasonings, and baking items

- Salt and pepper
- Dry herbs: basil, bay leaves, oregano, parsley, tarragon, thyme, dill
- Spices: chili powder, ground cinnamon, paprika, dried mustard, ginger, curry
- Garlic powder, onion salt, celery salt
- Granulated and brown sugar
- Vanilla extract

- Bread or Cornflake crumbs
- Unbleached flour
- Honey

Produce Staples

- Potatoes
- Onions

Other stuff (space providing)

- Teabags
- Coffee
- Snack foods
- Crackers

FOR MORE INFORMATION . . .

Organizations/agencies

Food and Drug Administration (FDA)
 Center for Food Safety and Applied Nutrition
 800-FDA–4010
 www.cfsan.fda.gov

United States Department of Agriculture (USDA)
 Meat and Poultry Hotline
 800–535–4555
 www.fsis.usda.gov

CHART 12–12

Grocery List

Fresh Fruits and Vegetables
_____
_____

Dairy
Milk, Yogurt, Cheese
_____
_____
_____

Frozen Foods
Vegetables
_____
_____
_____

Grain Foods
Bread, Bagels, English muffins, Pasta, Cereal
_____
_____
_____

Canned and Packaged Food
Soup, Tuna fish
_____
_____
_____

Bottled and Jarred Food
_____
_____
_____

Other Stuff
_____
_____
_____

Boiling Water 101

If you don't know how to boil water, the thought of cooking an entire meal may seem entirely out of your reach. You're not alone. Many people avoid cooking because it looks like too much trouble or think it takes too much time. With a "drive thru" on every corner, do you even need to learn to cook? You probably do.

There are lots of good reasons to get comfortable in the kitchen:

- Fast foods and eating out get old and monotonous after a while.
- Eating out is expensive. Cooking your own meals is **a lot** cheaper.
- You can choose what to eat and when.
- What you prepare can be fresh, healthful, delicious, and easy to make.
- Cooking can be fun.

A kitchen may seem intimidating if you haven't cooked much. Adopt a new attitude. Think of the kitchen as your science lab. Just as you perform experiments by following the steps in a science book, you can prepare food following the steps in a recipe book.

However, before you venture off to create your first masterpiece, take time to learn the language (see Chart 13–6 at the end of this chapter) and a few of the ground rules for making sure your food is safe and tasty.

Keep your Kitchen Clean.

Your kitchen is like a petri dish. It's the perfect environment for bacteria to flourish, some of which can be harmful. Bacteria can be responsible for a whole host of problems, from mild diarrhea to death (in rare situations). You can greatly minimize your risk of food poisoning by keeping your kitchen clean (see Chapter 12).

- Start with clean hands.

  Wash them well with soap and hot water before you touch food and after you handle raw meat.

- Keep surfaces clean.

  Food contains bacteria, as do the surfaces with which food comes in contact. Always keep cutting boards and countertops clean. Wash dishtowels frequently; replace sponges and dishcloths often.

- Avoid transferring bacteria from one place to another.

  Once you've started preparing food, clean surfaces and utensils between each step. For example, after you dice the veggies, wash utensils and cutting boards/countertops before cutting up meat.

Treating raw meat, poultry, and fish properly is especially important. As soon as you get home from grocery shopping, refrigerate or freeze these foods. To limit the transfer of bacteria from food to food, be sure meat is placed in a plastic bag or on a plate in the refrigerator so none of its juices will come in contact with other foods. Ideally, purchase two cutting boards and use one for cutting meat and one for cutting everything else. After cutting chicken or meat, be sure to wash the knife and the cutting boards thoroughly in hot, soapy water.

Store foods carefully.

Storing foods properly is an art and a science. The art is figuring out how to store food given your limited space. The science is knowing how to store food to keep it fresh and safe to eat. If you open a can of food, such as soup or tuna fish, and plan to save part of it, transfer the leftover portion to a non-metal container before refrigerating it. If you don't, the metallic taste of the can is absorbed by the food, giving it an off flavor.

If you have leftover cooked food, wrap and store it in the refrigerator as well. Let it cool slightly before you place it in the refrigerator. Putting hot food directly into the refrigerator can cause the temperature to rise in the refrigerator. Leftovers should always be reheated thoroughly before eating.

Don't let perishable food sit out on the counter for more than two hours. The bacteria that causes food poisoning thrives at room temperature. Pay attention to the timetable for keeping food safe. **When in doubt, throw it out**.

Handle Cutlery with Care

Knives, whether sharp or dull, are potential hazards in the kitchen. Always pick up a knife by its handle, not its blade. Don't throw it into a sink full of dirty dishes; it can get lost under the pile and you can cut yourself when you wash the dishes. Instead, wash knives separately, then return them to a safe storage space.

To avoid injury, always use a cutting board when cutting anything with a knife. Like knives, vegetable peelers are sharp. When peeling potatoes, carrots, or cucumbers, peel in a direction away from your body. This is safer and a more efficient movement.

Respect the Stove and Oven

If food burns, and it will, take simple precautions not to burn yourself or others. Always use oven mitts and potholders when removing dishes from the oven, stove, or microwave. Should a fire start on top of the stove or in the oven, remove the pot or pan from the heat, if possible. Try to shut off the air supply to the fire by closing the oven door or putting a lid on the pot. Remember that water and oil do not mix, so dousing flames with water may not work and can actually make matters worse. Instead, keep a box of baking soda near the stove and pour it on the fire if the fire doesn't seem out of control. If you sense the flames may be getting out of control, call the fire department.

When cooking, turn all pot and pan handles toward the center of the stove so they don't stick out and snag someone walking by. Avoid wearing long, flowing sleeves, such as on a bathrobe or some shirts when you cook. They can easily get caught on cooking handles or touch a flame.

Things spill, boil over, or drip while you're cooking. As soon as the cooktop has cooled off, wipe up the mess. Wiping up spills as they occur is much less work than trying to chisel off dried-up, crusted-over mishaps from last week.

Put Stuff Back Where You Got It

Being a neatness freak may not be your forte, but if you make an effort to put things back in their proper place, you'll have a much easier time with the entire kitchen experience. No one expects to walk into a perfectly organized kitchen, but you can avoid a lot of hassles and frustrations when you find space for everything you use and stick to using that space.

Have a Game Plan

Read a recipe from beginning to end before you start making it (see Chart 13–1). Make sure you have all of the ingredients and equipment you need, and that you have enough time to adequately prepare the recipe. Although you'll eventually be comfortable improvising with

---

CHART 13–1

Common Cooking Abbreviations

Abbreviation	What it means
c./C.	cup
lb.	pound
ml.	milliliter
oz.	ounce
pt.	pint
t./tsp.	teaspoon
T. /TB. / Tbs./Tbsp.	Tablespoon

ingredients, making banana bread without bananas will never fly (see Chart 13–2 and 13–3).

Don't be a Slave to Recipes

It pays to follow a recipe as written the first time you use it. As you gain confidence and experience, you can make changes and adaptations. As you become more comfortable, experiment with substitutions that make sense to you. For instance, if something calls for lime but you don't have a lime, use a lemon. Think about the flavors that appeal to

CHART 13–2

Substituting Ingredients

If the recipe says . . .	It means . . .
1 glove of garlic	⅛ teaspoon of garlic powder
1 tablespoon of fresh herbs	1 teaspoon of dried herbs
1 teaspoon of dried mustard	1 tablespoon of prepared mustard
1 cup of sour cream	1 cup of plain yogurt
2 cups of fresh tomatoes	2 cups of canned tomatoes
1 cup of buttermilk	1 cup of warm skim milk plus 1 tablespoon of vinegar or lemon juice, or 1 cup of plain yogurt
¾ cup cracker crumbs	1 cup bread crumbs

CHART 13–3

Common Recipe Conversions

If the recipe says . . .	It means . . .
1 pound of bananas or apples	3 medium bananas or apples
2 tablespoons of butter	¼ stick of butter
6 ounces of chocolate chips	¼ cup of chocolate chips
½ pound of cheese	2 cups of pre-shredded cheese
1 medium lemon	3 tablespoons of lemon juice
1 large onion	1 cup chopped onion
2 ounces of nuts	⅓ cup chopped nuts
½ pound or 2 cups uncooked pasta	4 cups cooked pasta
pinch or dash of seasoning	less than ⅛ teaspoon
3 teaspoons	1 tablespoon
2 tablespoons	1 fluid ounce
4 tablespoons	¼ cup
1 cup	8 fluid ounces
2 cups	1 pint
2 pints	1 quart
4 quarts	1 gallon

you. If you're a salsa person, try using it as a sauce on fish and chicken. Before you know it, you'll have created your own recipes.

Seasoned cooks generally rely on six or eight recipes which they vary to make new dishes. Once you've mastered three recipes, you're on your way to self-sufficiency.

Have Fun

Go for it and get adventurous in the kitchen. All you need are a few basic cooking skills, a handful of recipes to get you going, and some time to experiment.

Cooking Techniques: Skills to Master

You'll need to become familiar with a whole vocabulary of cooking and a host of tricks to reduce your learning curve. These helpful hints can teach you how to think and act like a true chef.

Chopping an Onion

Using a sharp knife and a cutting board, cut stem ends off onion. Peel off outer skin. Cut onion in half lengthwise. Place onion halves on cutting board with the cut side facing down. Cut onion halves lengthwise into strips. Then cut across strips, making small chunks.

Cooking until Done

This vague direction assumes you've made this dish before. "Doneness" is relative. What may seem fine to you may seem overcooked to your roommate. Undercooking foods may be acceptable for veggies or pasta if you prefer them "al dente," but it can be downright dangerous

---

CHART 13–4

Testing for Doneness

POULTRY: Cut a small slit in the thickest part of the meat. The juice running out should be clear, not pink. When in doubt, cook the food ten minutes longer.

BEEF: Use the "touch test." Remove the meat from the oven and touch it. If it's done, it should bounce back slightly when touched. If it doesn't, cook it a few more minutes. Like poultry, you can always cut the meat in the thickest part. If it's slightly pink, it's ready to eat. Really red requires a few more minutes of cooking. Be sure to cook ground beef thoroughly. Rare may taste good, but it isn't safe to eat.

FISH: Use your eyes for this one. Raw fish changes color; it goes from translucent to milky white or opaque when done. When you cut cooked fish, it should be flaky. You can also apply the "fish rule"-cook fish ten minutes for every inch of thickness.

PASTA AND NOODLES: Taste a piece; it should be soft, not crunchy.

RICE: All of the cooking liquid should be absorbed.

VEGETABLES: These can be eaten raw, crunchy, or cooked. The exceptions are potatoes, Brussels sprouts, and artichokes, which need to be cooked before eating. Potatoes should be soft to the touch. You should be able to remove the outer leaves from artichokes and Brussel sprouts easily.

when it comes to poultry, pork, and beef. Meat thermometers take the guesswork out of cooking because they are labeled with the correct cooking temperatures for large cuts of meat, such as roasts, whole turkeys and chicken. Chances are you're not feeding an army, just cooking for one or two. Therefore, there are other ways you can check the doneness besides using a thermometer (see Chart 13–4).

Testing for doneness gets easier with practice. If you undercook a food, you can always correct it by putting it in the microwave (if you have one) or back in the oven. It may affect the texture of what you are cooking, however. But, as they say, better safe than sorry.

Cracking Eggs

Tap the egg gently on the side of a dish or the counter. Using your fingers, pull the shell apart at the crack, allowing the egg to drop into a bowl.

Defrosting Foods

Breads, cakes, cookies, and other baked goods can be defrosted by leaving them on the kitchen counter at room temperature. Meats, poultry, fish, and casserole dishes such as lasagna should be defrosted in the refrigerator. Defrosting at room temperature is not recommended for these foods because bacteria grow rapidly at room temperature, making the food unsafe to eat. Be sure to allow 24–36 hours to defrost a food thoroughly. An alternative is to defrost items using the microwave. If you do, cook items promptly after defrosting them.

Greasing a Pan

Put a small amount of butter, margarine, or oil on a paper towel and spread it on the bottom and side of pans. You can also use your clean fingers. Cooking sprays can often be substituted.

Measuring

Measure all ingredients in a recipe. The success of baked goods like cakes, cookies, and breads depend on it, as do many of the other dishes

you'll make. Measure over the sink or counter instead of your working bowl or pot, since it may already have measured ingredients in it.
Then, if you make a mistake and pour too much, you won't ruin the
entire dish (see Chart 13–5).

CHART 13–5

How to Measure

You need three basic measuring tools:

- **A glass or plastic measuring cup** with a spout for pouring,
- **A set of plastic or metal measuring cups**, which usually includes
  a 1 cup, ½ cup, ⅓ cup, and ¼ cup, and
- **A set of spoons** which includes 1 tablespoon, 1 teaspoon,
  ½ teaspoon and ¼ teaspoon.

**Dry ingredients such as flour, sugar, and rice are measured with the
plastic measuring cups.** The correct technique is to dip the measuring
cup into the container of flour (or other ingredient) and scoop out more
than you need. Using the edge of a knife, level off the top. Always work
over a plate or paper to catch the overflow. When measuring brown
sugar, be sure to mash out the lumps before you measure. (To prevent
it from hardening, brown sugar should be stored in a ziplock bag or
airtight container.)

Measuring cups are also used for portioning solid fats, such as tub
margarine or butter. Stick butter has measurements pre-printed on the
paper wrapper thereby eliminating the need to use a spoon or cup to
measure it. When measuring tub margarine or butter, let it sit at room
temperature for about 30 minutes so it will soften. It will be much easier to
scoop into a measuring tool. As with dry ingredients, measure more than
needed into the measuring cup and level it off with the edge of a knife.

**Liquids such as water, milk, or juice are measured in the spouted
measuring cup.** Place the cup on a level surface such as a table or
countertop. Slowly pour liquid into the measuring cup, bending down to
check the measurement marker rather than holding the cup at eye level.

**Measuring spoons are used to measure small amounts of liquids
such as vanilla extract and dry ingredients such as seasonings.** For
dry measuring, again, dip the spoon into the seasoning box and use
a knife to level off the ingredients. If the recipe calls for a "heaping
tablespoonful," it means to use as much as one tablespoon can hold.

Preheating

Many recipes ask you to preheat the oven. If you're rushed, you may not always have the time, or you may simply forget to do it. Preheating the oven affects the outcome of certain foods. As a rule of thumb, you should always preheat an oven when baking cakes, bread, pies, cookies, and some pizzas, or when you are roasting meat or poultry. Preheating is generally not necessary if you're heating leftovers.

Seasoning

Seasoning is an art. To do it right, you need to taste as you cook and add seasonings along the way. Use a steady hand; you can always increase the amount you put in, but you can never subtract what you've added. If the recipe says "season to taste," start with a small amount. After you've eaten the finished product, write notes to remember your changes or additions.

Separating an Egg

Crack the egg as directed. Pull the shell apart carefully at the crack then transfer the yolk between the halves, allowing the egg white to fall out.

Washing Lettuce

Pull apart the amount of lettuce you want to eat. Rinse it under water and pat dry with a clean paper towel or dishtowel. A salad spinner is available to do this job, but it can be done easily without one.

Cooking Techniques: On the Stove

Boiling

Boiling occurs when water reaches 212 degrees. A **full** or **rolling boil** is when the bubbles break the surface of the water. Covering a pot and adding a small amount of salt helps the liquid come to a boil more quickly. Typically, rice, pasta, and potatoes are boiled in large amounts of water. Once boiled foods are cooked, the recipe will instruct you to **drain** the foods. This means getting rid of the cooking water while retaining the cooked food. Use a **colander** to accomplish this. Place the colander in the sink and pour the entire contents of the pan (food and liquid) into the colander, letting the liquid drain.

Simmering

To keep the food at a boiling temperature but having the bubbles barely break the surface is known as simmering. This is done by keeping the heat or flame lower than used for boiling. Soups, stews, and casseroles generally are simmered.

Poaching

One step under a simmer is poaching. The heat is on high enough to see the bubbles, but they don't break the surface of the liquid.

Steaming

Steaming food is accomplished by using a small amount of simmering water. The pan is often covered to keep the steam from escaping. To steam foods easily, you can purchase a small metal steamer. If using a steamer, add a small amount of water to a saucepan, place the steamer in the saucepan, put vegetables in the steamer, and cover. Vegetables and fish can be steamed or poached.

Sautéing and Stir-frying

These two terms are the same. Sautéing is a French term meaning "jumps," which is what food does when it is sautéed. You actually make it jump by stirring it quickly in a hot pan or wok on top of the stove using a small amount of cooking oil, spray, or fat. You hear the food cook by the crackling sounds it makes. You need to watch the food carefully so it doesn't stick to the pan and burn. Meats, poultry, fish, and veggies can all be sautéed.

Frying

Frying is a cooking technique in which food is immersed in a large quantity of hot oil. Frying food on a regular basis isn't a healthy way to prepare it and is impractical for most college cooking situations.

Cooking Techniques: The Oven and Broiler

Baking and Roasting

Both baking and roasting are done behind a closed oven door. Foods are cooked by dry heat circulating in the oven. The key to success is an accurate oven temperature. It's quite possible the oven you have is past its prime, and its temperature may be off a bit. When you first use the oven, note whether cooking times given for a recipe coincide with how your oven is performing. As you become more comfortable making meals, you may note that your oven cooks faster or slower than the suggested times in recipes and you can make adjustments accordingly.

Generally, **baking is used for cookies, cake, breads,** and **pies** and for preparing **chicken** and **fish**. Meat is rarely baked. **Roasting** is done at a higher heat and is an appropriate method for cooking **meat, poultry,** and **vegetables**. Bake or roast foods in the middle of the oven unless the recipe states otherwise.

Sometimes a recipe that calls for baked or roasted foods will require you to **baste** as well. Basting means to spoon juices over cooked meat. This is done to keep meat moist and tender. Basting is done by brushing the dripping juices from a meat with a small brush or using a spoon and pouring juices from the roasting pan back over the cooking meat. You can also purchase a bulb baster that allows you to suck up the juices at the bottom of a pan, then squeeze them back over the cooked meat.

Grilling and Broiling

These techniques are essentially the same cooking procedure. The main difference is that in grilling, the heat source is below the food. In broiling, the heat source is above the food. If you have an electric oven, the broiler is the upper heating coil in your oven. In a gas oven, it's a flame found below the oven. Toaster ovens generally have a broiler option, too.

It's best to broil foods on a broiling pan. This type of pan has a grated top with holes in it that allow juices from meat to drip into the holding pan below. When broiling, place a broiler pan about four inches from the heat source. To prevent cleanup hassles, line the bottom of the pan with aluminum foil so you can toss it out when you are done cooking.

Almost any food can be grilled or broiled. Most often, you will broil **thick cuts of meat, chicken, fish,** and **some vegetables**. Thicker cuts of meat will take slightly longer to broil than thin ones. Since food is being cooked very close to the heat source, it usually doesn't take long. You must watch foods carefully to ensure they don't burn.

Cooking Techniques: The Microwave

Although technically microwaving is not a cooking technique, the microwave is one of the most commonly used cooking methods for students. Microwave cooking occurs when microwaves agitate the water molecules in a food, causing them to heat up, which, in turn, heats up the food. For this to happen, the food in the microwave must be in a **microwave-safe** container. Aluminum foil should never be used in a microwave oven (see Chapter 12).

Most people rely on the microwave to reheat or **nuke** foods or to **defrost** (thaw out) frozen foods. Actually, many foods lend themselves to microwave cooking. Baked potatoes cook well in a microwave. **Chicken, fish,** and **vegetables** do also; however, when cooked in a microwave, they won't "brown" the same way they do when cooked in a conventional oven. With certain modifications, you can even bake cookies and cakes in a microwave. There are several recipe books specifically for microwave cooking.

Cooking time in a microwave oven is generally less than cooking time in a conventional oven. Cutting foods into smaller pieces speeds up the cooking process, as does covering dishes. When cooking in a microwave, be sure to rotate or turn foods often to ensure a more even distribution of heat.

A word of caution. Although the microwave oven itself does not emit heat, the food you cook does. When taking foods out of a micro-wave, always use an oven mitt or potholder. Also, when unwrapping a container or taking off a cover, don't put your face or hands near the top. The steam escaping from the cooked dish can cause serious burns.

From Ingredients to Table

Having everything hit the table at the correct temperature at the same time takes practice. When planning a meal, consider the prepara-tion and cooking time of each dish. For instance, don't make one dish that requires 30 minutes at 450° and one that takes 60 minutes at 350° if you have one oven.

Initially, choose one main course and serve it with a simple salad. Once you've got that mastered, add steamed veggies, potato or another type of side dish. Make salads and room temperature dishes first. Cover them and refrigerate until you are ready to eat. Right before serving, add dressing if desired.

Great-tasting, healthy meals can come out of a makeshift dorm room kitchen or full-size kitchen. It's a matter of organization and experience. Choose simple recipes to start. Make sure you have plenty of time to prepare, cook, and clean up. Then, invite a friend or two and enjoy being self-sufficient.

CHART 13–6

Glossary of Common Cooking Terms

AL DENTE: An Italian term, literally meaning "to the tooth," used to describe the texture of food, usually pasta, which is cooked, but still firm.

BAKE: To cook, covered or uncovered, by dry heat in the oven. Cakes, cookies, pies, and casseroles are baked.

BARBECUE: To cook on a gas or charcoal grill.

BASTE: To add moisture and flavor to food by brushing on or adding to the food seasoned liquid, fat, or drippings.

BATTER: A liquid mixture usually containing flour and other ingredients that can be dropped from a spoon or poured.

BEAT: To stir or mix with a machine, spoon, or whisk, adding air to make the mixture light and smooth.

BLANCH: To boil vegetables or fruit for a short time to remove or loosen their skins or preserve their color.

BLEND: To completely mix together two or more ingredients using a spoon, fork spatula, whisk, or blender.

BOIL: To bring liquid to a temperature of 212° allowing large bubbles to rise and break the surface.

BRAISE: To cook foods slowly in a small amount of liquid, either on the stove or in the oven. Chicken and meat are often braised.

BREAD: To coat foods with crackers, breadcrumbs, or cracker crumbs to seal in moisture in preparation for frying or baking. Food is first dipped in beaten eggs, milk, or other liquid to allow the crumbs to adhere to the food.

BROIL: To cook by intense direct heat under a hot oven coil, either in a broiler or a toaster oven.

BROWN: To cook the outside of food quickly over high heat on top of the stove to seal in flavor.

CHOP: To cut food into small pieces.

CORE: To remove the center of a fruit or vegetable.

CUBE: To cut food into cube-shaped pieces that are the same size.

DASH: A small amount of any ingredient.

DEBONE: To remove the bones from fish, poultry, or beef.

DICE: To cut into very small pieces of the same size and shape.

DRAIN: To remove the liquid from a food, usually by pouring the food into a colander and letting the liquid drain through the holes.

DREDGE: To coat the outside of food with a dry ingredient, such as flour, crackers, or breadcrumbs.

FILLET: To remove the bones from a piece of fish or meat. Fillet is also used to describe the piece of fish or meat after the bones have been removed.

FOLD: To combine a lighter mixture, such as beaten egg whites with a heavier mixture, such as egg yolks and sugar, using a gentle over-and-under motion.

FRY: To cook food in hot oil in an open skillet or frying pan. Submerging food in the fat is deep-frying the food.

GRATE: To cut food into very fine pieces or shreds by rubbing it against a metal utensil with serrated holes called a grater, or using an electric food processor.

GREASE: To rub oil, margarine, or butter onto the bottom and sides of a baking sheet or pan to prevent food from sticking.

GRILL: To cook food on a rack directly over the heat source.

GRIND: To chop food very finely with a food grinder or in a food processor.

JULIENNE: To cut food into matchstick-size strips.

KNEAD: To work dough with hands until it becomes smooth and elastic.

MARINATE: To soak foods in a seasoned liquid for several hours or overnight in the refrigerator to make it more tender and flavorful.

MINCE: To cut or chop food into tiny pieces.

MIX: To combine two or more ingredients until blended well.

PARBOIL: To cook food in boiling water for a very short time.

PARE: To remove the skin or peel from fruits or vegetables.

PINCH: A very small amount of any dry ingredient.

POACH: To cook foods in barely boiling water. Eggs and fish are often poached.

POUND: To flatten foods, such as chicken breasts, with a mallet to an even thickness.

PREHEAT: To heat the oven to the desired temperature before beginning to cook.

PUREE: To mash or blend to a smooth consistency.

ROAST: To cook in the hot, dry heat of an oven. Meat and chicken are often roasted.

SAUTÉ: To cook food quickly over high heat in a small amount of butter or fat.

SEAR:	To brown meat quickly by cooking over high heat, in the broiler, or in a very hot oven to seal in flavor and moisture.
SEASON:	To flavor foods using salt, pepper, herbs, and spices.
SHRED:	To cut food into thin, irregular strips usually using a grater or food processor.
SIFT:	To pass flour or other dry ingredients through a sieve or sifter before measuring to remove lumps.
SIMMER:	To cook food in liquid just below the boiling point.
STEAM:	To cook food using the water vapor from boiling water in a covered pot or a metal basket that fits into a pot. Vegetables and fish can be steamed.
STEW:	To cook food by slowly simmering in a small amount of liquid in a covered pot.
STIR:	To mix ingredients without beating using a spoon.
STIR-FRY:	To cook cut-up food quickly in a small amount of oil or liquid by stirring constantly over high heat. Stir-frying can be done in a frying pan or wok.
STOCK:	The liquid left over from cooking meat, fish, poultry, or vegetables, often used as a base for soups and sauces.
STRAIN:	To separate solid ingredients from the liquid they have been cooked in by pouring them through a colander or sieve.
TOSS:	To mix ingredients gently by lifting and turning with two spoons, forks, or your hands. Salad and pasta are often tossed.
WHIP:	To beat air into ingredients using a whisk or mixer, making them light and fluffy.

CHAPTER

14

Recipes

The following recipes are "starters." The number of recipes offered here is intentionally limited. Too many recipes seem to paralyze people. Most of these recipes are for main courses only. To make a complete meal, buy salad ingredients, steam plain vegetables, or cut up fruit. If the main courses you choose do not include rice, pasta, or potatoes, add a simple grain such as a slice of bread.

Portions are for average servings and most serve four people. Most of these recipes can be easily doubled to serve more people.

Feel free to experiment with ingredients. Add some extra sauce or eliminate a seasoning. Be sure to write down your own modifications. As you discover the joys of cooking, you may want to explore cookbooks. Walk into a bookstore and you will find literally hundreds of inviting cookbooks. To give you a head start, those listed at the end of this section are in the category of "simple," "healthy," or "quick."

No Cook Main Dishes

EGGLESS SALAD

1 pkg. (10.5 or 12 oz.) firm tofu	1 Tbsp. sugar
	1 Tbsp. mustard
¼ cup chopped celery (or ½ tsp. celery seed)	2 Tbsp. vinegar
	Black pepper to taste
¼ cup green or red pepper	½ tsp. salt
2 Tbsp. finely chopped green onion (or ½ tsp. onion powder)	

1. Drain tofu and crumble into a bowl.
2. Combine the honey, mustard, vinegar, black pepper, salt (and onion powder/celery seed) in a small cup.
3. Pour over tofu and mix well.
4. Add celery, pepper and onion.

SERVES 4

Per serving: 140 calories, 14 gm protein, 8 gm carbohydrate, 7 gm fat

BEAN BURRITOS

4 flour tortillas	½ cup salsa
1 can (16 oz.) vegetarian refried beans	½ cup shredded cheddar cheese

1. Divide beans between tortillas.
2. Top with salsa and cheese.
3. Roll tortilla, tucking in at the end.
4. If you have a microwave, you can heat these on high for one minute and the cheese will melt.

SERVES 4

Per serving: 340 calories, 15 gm protein, 49 gm carbohydrate, 10 gm fat

Corn and Bean Salad

1 can (15 oz.) whole kernel corn, drained
1 can (15 oz.) black beans, drained
4 scallions, chopped
1 green pepper, diced
1 cup salsa

1. Combine corn, beans, scallions, green pepper.
2. Add salsa.

SERVES 4

Per serving: 237 calories, 12 gm protein, 48 gm carbohydrate, 2 gm fat

Tomato and Cheese Salad

2 medium tomatoes, sliced
2 oz. part-skim mozzarella cheese, cut in thin slices
2 Tbsp. vinegar
1 Tbsp. olive oil
Salt and pepper

1. Place slice of cheese on tomato.
2. Drizzle with vinegar, oil and seasoning.

SERVES 4

Per serving: 72 calories, 4 gm protein, 2 gm carbohydrate, 6 gm fat

Three Bean Salad

1 can (15 oz.) kidney beans, drained
1 can (15 oz.) garbanzo beans, drained
1 can (15 oz.) green beans, drained
¼ cup red wine, balsamic or rice vinegar
1 Tbsp. parsley
¼ tsp. onion powder
¼ tsp. garlic powder

1. Combine beans in a large bowl.
2. Add remaining ingredients and mix well.

SERVES 4–6

Per larger serving: 270 calories, 17 gm protein, 50 gm carbohydrate, 1 gm fat

Veggie Rollups

4 large flour tortillas	4 scallions, chopped
½ cup hummus or 4 oz. feta cheese, crumbled	1 cup lettuce, shredded
	½ cucumber, chopped

1. Divide hummus or cheese on tortilla.
2. Top with veggies.
3. Roll up tortillla.

SERVES 4

Per serving: 294 calories, 8 gm protein, 48 gm carbohydrate, 8 gm fat

Asian Tofu Salad

1 pkg. (10.5 or 12 oz.) firm tofu	¼ tsp. ginger powder
2 scallions, chopped	¼ tsp. garlic powder
½ green or red pepper, chopped	1 Tbsp. honey
3 Tbsp. soy sauce	1 Tbsp. dry mustard

1. Drain tofu and crumble into a bowl.
2. Combine soy sauce, ginger powder, garlic powder, honey, and mustard.
3. Pour over tofu and mix well.
4. Add onions and pepper.

SERVES 4

Per serving: 105 calories, 8 gm protein, 10 gm carbohydrate, 5 gm fat

Fish, Poultry, and Meat

LEMON FISH

1 **lb. mild fish fillets such as orange roughy, flounder, or cod**	1½ **tsp. fresh lemon juice**
½ **cup bread crumbs**	1 **Tbsp. parsley**
2 **Tbsp. butter or margarine**	**Salt and pepper**

1. Rinse fillets and pat dry with paper towel.
2. Sprinkle fish with salt and pepper.
3. Place fish in microwave-safe dish.
4. Melt butter, either on top of stove over low heat or in microwave.
5. Add breadcrumbs, lemon juice, and parsley to melted butter.
6. Sprinkle mixture on top of fish.
7. Cover dish with saran wrap, if using the microwave.
8. Bake at 350° for about 10 minutes or microwave for 5–7 minutes.

SERVES 4

Per serving: 208 calories, 23 gm protein, 10 gm carbohydrate, 8 gm fat

COMPANY POACHED FISH

1 **lb. Salmon, orange roughy, or other fillets**	¼ **tsp. Garlic powder or 1 clove, minced**
1 **red pepper, cut in strips**	2 **Tbsp. soy sauce**
½ **onion chopped**	1 **Tbsp. olive oil**
6 **mushrooms, sliced**	**Silver foil, large enough to wrap around each fillet**
1 **Tbsp. lemon juice**	

1. Place each fish fillet on a piece of foil.
2. Divide veggies over each fish fillet.
3. In a small bowl, combine lemon juice, soy sauce, garlic and olive oil. Pour it evenly over fillets.
4. Close foil around fillet.
5. Bake in oven at 350° for about 20 minutes.

SERVES 4

Per serving: 259 calories, 23 gm protein, 4 gm carbohydrate, 16 gm fat

PLAIN BAKED CHICKEN

4   boneless, skinless chicken   Salt, pepper, garlic
     breasts*   powder, paprika
Nonstick spray oil or 1-2
Tbsp. olive oil

1. Coat bottom of glass baking dish with olive oil. Then rub
    some oil on chicken breasts to prevent them from drying out.
2. Sprinkle breasts with seasonings.
3. Bake in oven at 350° for 30 minutes or microwave
    for 12–15 minutes.

SERVES 4

Per serving: 140 calories, 26 gm protein, 0 gm carbohydrate, 3 gm fat

* You can use breasts with bone and skin. If the breasts have skin, there is no need to oil
them. Bake chicken pieces 45-60 minutes if they have a bone.

OVEN FRIED CHICKEN

4   boneless, skinless chicken   ½   cup cornflakes, crumbled
     breasts   Nonstick spray or 2 Tbsp.
¼   cup skim milk   olive oil
½   cup grated Parmesan   Salt and pepper
     cheese

1. Coat the bottom of a glass baking dish with nonstick spray or
    olive oil.
2. Combine the crumbs and cheese in a small bowl.
3. Dip chicken breasts in milk and then the cheese mixture.
4. Place chicken in dish.
5. Bake at 350° for 30 minutes, turning every 10 minutes, or
    microwave for 12–15 minutes.

SERVES 4

Per serving: 214 calories, 32 gm protein, 4 gm carbohydrate, 7 gm fat

Barbecued Chicken Breasts

4 boneless, skinless chicken breasts
¼ cup orange juice
½ cup prepared barbecue sauce

⅛ tsp. black pepper
Nonstick spray or 1 Tbsp. olive oil

1. Cut chicken breasts in long, narrow strips.
2. Combine orange juice, barbecue sauce, and black pepper.
3. Heat oil in frying pan or spray with nonstick spray.
4. Add chicken and stir-fry for about 10 minutes, until chicken looks cooked.
5. Add sauce and heat until it boils.

SERVES 4

Per serving: 170 calories, 27 gm protein, 5.5 gm carbohydrate, 4 gm fat

Apricot Chicken

4 boneless, skinless chicken breasts
½ cup flour
¼ tsp. black pepper
Large ziplock bag

Nonstick spray or 2 Tbsp. olive oil
½ cup apricot preserves
1 Tbsp. Dijon mustard
½ cup nonfat, plain yogurt

1. Preheat oven to 375°.
2. Pour flour and pepper in plastic bag. Add chicken, reseal bag, and shake well until chicken is coated with flour.
3. Combine preserves, mustard, and yogurt in small bowl. Set aside.
4. Coat bottom of baking pan with spray or oil.
5. Place chicken in pan and bake for 20 minutes.
6. Spread preserves mixture over chicken. Continue cooking for 25 minutes.

SERVES 4

Per serving: 262 calories, 30 gm protein, 27 gm carbohydrate, 3 gm fat

SIMPLE SAUCES FOR BONELESS CHICKEN BREASTS OR FISH FILLETS

Add any of the following to cooked chicken or fish fillets for a more "elegant" meal. One recipe should "top" 4 pieces of fish or chicken.

Mexican Style

1. Squeeze fresh lemon or lime juice over chicken or fish.
2. Heat 1 cup of salsa in microwave or in small pan on stove.
3. Top each piece of chicken or fish with salsa.

Per serving: 12 calories, .5 gm protein, 3 gm carbohydrate, 0 fat

Pepper Sauce

1. Sauté 5 chopped scallions and 1 Tbsp. minced garlic or garlic powder in 1 Tbsp. olive oil.
2. Add one 8 oz. jar of red pepper.
3. Heat through. Pour over chicken or fish.

Per serving: 41 calories, .5 gm protein, 2 gm carbohydrate, 4 gm fat

FABULOUS FLANK STEAK

1½	lb. flank steak	½	cup soy sauce
1	large onion, sliced	3	Tbsp. olive oil
1	cup mushrooms, sliced		Pepper

1. Sprinkle steak with pepper.
2. Put sliced onion and mushrooms over steak in large dish.
3. Mix soy sauce and olive oil.
4. Pour over steak. Cover with saran wrap and place in the refrigerator to marinate for at least 6 hours.
5. Lift steak from marinade and broil steak for about 4 minutes on each side.
6. While the steak is broiling, boil the marinade and vegetables. Reduce heat and simmer. Pour over cooked meat.

SERVES 4

Per serving: 304 calories, 32 gm protein, 3 gm carbohydrate, 17 gm fat

CHILI

1	lb. of ground beef or ground turkey	½	tsp. garlic powder
1	onion, chopped	1	can (15 oz.) kidney beans, drained
1	green pepper, chopped	1	can (15 oz.) tomato sauce
1½	Tbsp. chili powder		Nonstick spray or 1 Tbsp. olive oil
½	tsp. salt		

1. Spray bottom of saucepan with cooking spray or heat olive oil over low heat.
2. Add onions and green pepper. Cook until they are soft.
3. Add ground meat. Stir constantly until it is brown.
4. Drain any liquid into an empty juice or milk carton.
5. Add kidney beans, tomato sauce, chili powder, garlic powder, salt and pepper to mixture. Stir well.
6. Cook until the mixture boils, stirring often.
7. Lower heat and let it simmer about 15 minutes.

SERVES 4

Per serving: 302 calories, 27 gm protein, 27 gm carbohydrate, 10 gm fat

Survival Basics

BASIC PASTA

Pasta comes with cooking instructions . . . but the following directions will make it impossible to ruin. If you are using pasta as the main course, one pound should easily feed 4-6 people.

1. Using the largest pot available, fill it with at least 4 quarts of water for 1 pound of pasta.
2. Bring the water to a boil. Add the pasta. Using a long fork, move the pasta in the water to separate the strands of pasta.
3. When the water returns to a boil, set a timer for the amount of minutes stated on the package of pasta.
4. After cooking the appropriate amount of time, check a piece of the cooked pasta by taking it out of the water and tasting it. It should be tender, not crunchy.
5. Drain the pasta by pouring it in a colander in the sink. It is now ready to serve.

SERVES 4–6

Per serving: 200 calories, 7 gm protein, 41 gm carbohydrate, 1 gm fat

BASIC RICE

1½   cup water, canned broth, or combination
1   cup long grain rice

1. Bring liquid to a boil.
2. Add rice.
3. Lower the heat and cover.
4. After 20 minutes, turn off the heat, but let the rice stand for another 15–20 minutes, covered.
5. Fluff the rice with a fork before serving.

SERVES 4–6

Per serving: 171 calories, 3 gm protein, 38 gm carbohydrate, 0 gm fat

Baked Potatoes

4 baking potatoes (Idaho is good for baking)

1. Preheat oven to 450°.
2. Scrub potatoes and pat dry.
3. Prick the potato all over with a fork.
4. Bake in center of oven, directly on oven rack for 45–60 minutes.

To microwave: follow steps 2 & 3.

5. Place potatoes on a paper towel in the microwave, arranging like spokes on a wheel.
6. Microwave on high for 12–15 minutes.

SERVES 4

Per serving: 220 calories, 4.5 gm protein, 51 gm carbohydrate, 0 gm fat

Hard-Cooked Eggs

4 eggs
water

1. Put eggs in sauce pan. Cover with water.
2. Heat water to a boil. Lower temperature and cover. Let simmer for 10 minutes.
3. Spill out hot water and run cold water over eggs. Refrigerate.

SERVES 4

Per serving: 74 calories, 6 gm protein, .5 gm carbohydrate, 5 gm fat

Egg Salad

4 hard-cooked eggs, with shell removed

Chopped celery and onion (optional)

4 Tbsp. mayonnaise

Salt and pepper

1. Place eggs in medium size bowl.
2. Chop into pieces.
3. Add mayonnaise. Mix well.
4. Add celery and onion. Mix well.
5. Season with salt and pepper.

SERVES 4

Per serving: 133 calories, 6 gm protein, 4 gm carbohydrate, 10 gm fat

Meatless Main Dishes

STEAMED OR STIR-FRIED VEGGIES

2 large onions, sliced

10 mushrooms, sliced

Nonstick spray or 1-2 Tbsp. olive oil

¼ cup soy sauce mixed with ¼ cup water or small can vegetable or chicken broth

Crumbled tofu (if desired)

1 10 oz. box of frozen broccoli, cauliflower, carrots, or combination

1. Sauté in large frying pan onions and mushrooms.
2. Add frozen vegetables, and sauté until they are soft.
2. Add liquid and heat through.

SERVES 4

Per serving: 54 calories, 3.5 gm protein, 11 gm carbohydrate, .5 gm fat

BAKED ZITI

15 oz. low-fat ricotta cheese

8 oz. part-skim shredded mozzarella cheese

1 lb. ziti

1 26 oz. or 32 oz. jar of spaghetti sauce

2 Tbsp. grated Parmesan cheese

1. Cook ziti as directed on box and drain well.
2. Combine ziti, ricotta, and mozzarella cheese.
3. Spread half of ziti mixture into bottom of a large casserole dish.
4. Pour 1 cup of sauce on top and sprinkle half of Parmesan cheese over it.
5. Repeat this layer.
6. Cover with foil for oven, plastic wrap for microwave oven.
7. Bake at 350° for 25 minutes, remove foil, and continue baking for another 15 minutes. Or, cover with plastic wrap and microwave for 10 minutes. Uncover, and microwave for an additional 5 minutes.

SERVES 6–8

Per small serving: 406 calories, 22 gm protein, 52 gm carbohydrate, 11 gm fat

Beans and Pasta

1	can (15oz.) of white canillini beans	10 oz. frozen spinach
2	cups cooked penne or rigatoni	Garlic powder, salt and pepper

1. Cook spinach as directed. Drain well.
2. Combine beans, pasta and spinach in medium size pot.
3. Season with garlic powder, salt and pepper.
4. Cook over low heat for about 10 minutes.

SERVES 4

Per serving: 278 calories, 13 gm protein, 43 gm carbohydrate, 7 gm fat

Scrambled Eggs

4 eggs	¼ cup skim milk
1 Tbsp. butter or margarine	salt and pepper

1. Crack eggs into medium size bowl.
2. Add milk. Whisk or mix with a fork until blended.
3. Put burner on a low heat. Melt butter in a frying pan over heat.
4. Pour egg mixture into pan. Let it sit for about 15 seconds.
5. Stir eggs gently with a fork, breaking up larger pieces. Sprinkle with salt and pepper. Serve immediately. Eggs should not be at all "runny".

SERVES 2

Per serving: 210 calories, 13.5 gm protein, 2.5 gm carbohydrate, 15 gm fat

PEANUT NOODLES

8 oz. uncooked pasta	¼ cup peanut butter
4 scallions, chopped	¼ cup soy sauce
1 cup of cooked peas, chopped carrots, celery, peppers or any leftover vegetables	1 Tbsp. oil
	½ tsp. Garlic powder
	¼ tsp. Black pepper

1. Cook pasta as directed.
2. Blend together peanut butter, soy sauce, oil, garlic powder and black pepper.
3. Drain pasta.
4. Pour sauce over pasta and add vegetables. Mix well.

SERVES 4

Per serving: 352 calories, 12 gm protein, 49 gm carbohydrate, 13 gm fat

CREATE-YOUR-OWN CASSEROLE

1. Choose one food from each of the columns.
2. Put all selected food in an ovenproof baking dish.
3. Place topping over food.
4. Bake uncovered at 350° for 25-30 minutes or microwave for 10-15 minutes.

BASE	VEGETABLES	SAUCE	MEAT	SEASONING	TPPING
2 cups cooked	1 cup cooked	1–2 cups	1 cup cooked	1 tsp.	1 cup
Noodles	Celery	Prepared	Ground beef	Chili powder	Grated,
Rice	Carrots	tomato	Ground	Garlic/	low fat
Pasta	Peas	sauce	turkey	onion	cheese
Couscous	Peppers	Chicken or	Chicken	powder	Bread
	Mushrooms	vegetable	Canned tuna	Pepper/salt	crumbs
	Green beans	stock			
	(Combination	Salsa			
	of above)	Soy sauce			

SERVES 4

Per serving: 215 calories, 17 gm protein, 22 gm carbohydrate, 6 gm fat

Snacks

PERSONAL PIZZA

1	English muffin	2	Tbsp. shredded
2	Tbsp. tomato or spaghetti sauce		mozzarella cheese

1. Split the English muffin into two halves.
2. Spread sauce evenly on both halves.
3. Sprinkle cheese evenly on both halves.
4. Broil in toaster oven for one minute or until cheese melts.

SERVES 1

Per serving: 234 calories, 13 gm protein, 32 gm carbohydrate, 7 gm fat

SMOOTHIES

½	carton vanilla yogurt	1	cup fruit
8	oz. fruit juice	4	ice cubes

1. Add all ingredients to a blender.
2. Blend until smooth.

SERVES 1

Per serving: 256 calories, 9 gm protein, 55 gm carbohydrate, 1 gm fat

FROZEN BANANA

1 banana

1. Peel banana.
2. Place on a plate covered with foil.
3. Place in freezer for at least 2 hours.

SERVES 1

Per serving: 108 calories, 1 gm protein, 28 gm carbohydrate, 0 gm fat

STEAMED EDAMAME (JAPANESE SOYBEANS)

1 bag of frozen edamame
¼ tsp. of salt

1. Boil salted water
2. Add edamame
3. Boil for 10 minutes.
4. Enjoy by eating the shell inside the bean.

Per ½ cup: 126 calories, 11g protein, 10g carbohydrates, 6g total fat

FOR MORE INFORMATION . . .

Books

Foco, Z. 1998. *Lickety-Split Meals.* Walled Lake, MI: ZHI.

Miller, B., and Rama., M. 1996. *Cooking for Dummies.* Foster City, CA. IDG Books Worldwide.

Nimetz, A., Stanley, J., and Starr, E. 1999. *The Healthy College Cookbook: Quick. Cheap. Easy.* North Adams, MA. Storey Publishing.

Ponichtera, B. 2005. *Quick & Healthy, Low-Fat, Carb Conscious Cooking.* 2nd Edition, The Dalles, OR. ScaleDown Publishing.

Index

Website Index

About the Author

Ann Selkowitz Litt, M.S., R.D., L.D. is a nutritionist who specializes in working with young adults and teenagers. (As the parent of two college students, she also has plenty of day-to-day experience with this age group.) In addition to private patient counseling, Ann is the nutritionist for **The Washington Redskins** and the author of *Fuel for Young Athletes* and *American Dietetic Association Guide to Private Practice*.

As an expert in healthy eating habits, Litt has been quoted in national publications including **The New York Times, The Washington Post**, and **The Wall Street Journal**. Ann has appeared on local and national television including the **CBS Morning Show** and the **NBC Later Today** show.

Professionally, Ann is highly regarded in the nutrition community. She is past chairperson of Nutrition Entrepreneurs, a Dietetic Practice Group of the American Dietetic Association, is a Professional Issues Delegate for Consultation and Business Practice in the American Dietetic Associations House of Delegates and was the recipient of the Recognized Young Dietitian Award from the ADA.

Order Form

TELEPHONE ORDERS: 301–229–1070
FAX ORDERS: 301–320–8595
WEBSITE: www.collegeeatingguide.com

MAIL ORDERS:
Tulip Hill Press
5257 River Road #305
Bethesda, MD 20816

Please send me_____copies of Eating Well on Campus
 @ 14.95 each* $_____

Shipping and Handling: $_____
  $4.50 per book; $1.00 for each additional book.

Maryland residents add 5% sales tax. $_____

Total enclosed $_____

Payment: ❏ Check   ❏ Visa   ❏ Mastercard

Card Number _____   Exp. Date_____

Name on card _____

SHIP TO:

Name _____

Address _____

_____

City _____   State_____   Zip _____

Telephone _____

*ll for quantity discount of more than 5 copies.